P9-DER-263

N A T U R A L
M E D I C I N E
FOR
WOMEN

2012
For my life's joy!
my Christene!
love,
mom

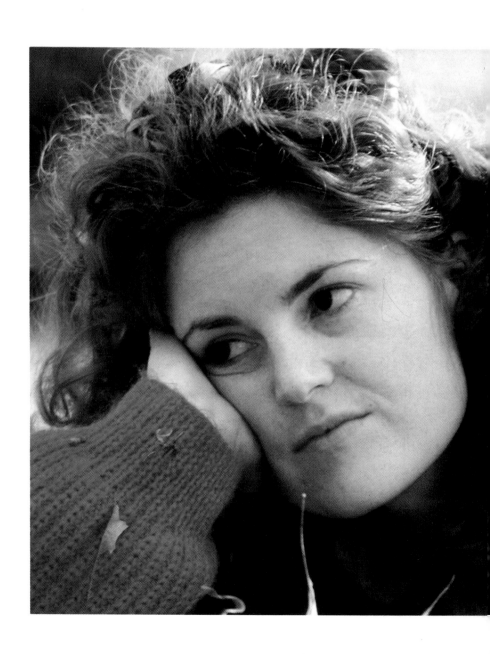

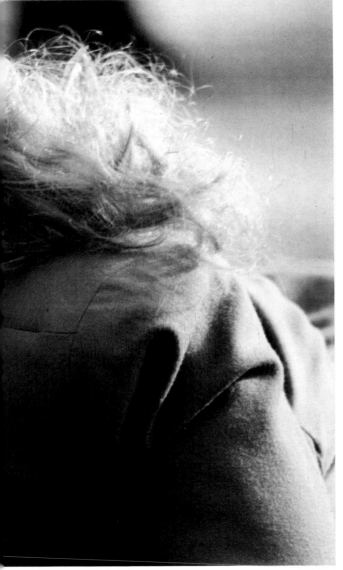

NATURAL MEDICINE FOR WOMEN

JULIAN AND SUSAN SCOTT

AVON BOOKS NEW YORK

A GAIA ORIGINAL

Editorial	Steve Parker
Design	Ellen Moorcraft
Illustration	Sheilagh Noble
Consultant	Robert Cran
Direction	Joss Pearson
	Patrick Nugent

Copyright © 1991 by Gaia Books
Text copyright © 1991 by Julian and Susan Scott

The right of Julian and Susan Scott to be identified as the authors of this work has been asserted in accordance with Sections 77 and 78 of the Copyright, Designs and Patents Act 1988, United Kingdom.

Printed and bound by Mateu Cromo, Madrid, Spain

AVON BOOKS
A division of
The Hearst Corporation
105 Madison Avenue
New York, New York 10016

Published by arrangement with Gaia Books Ltd

Library of Congress Catalog Card Number: 91-91874
ISBN: 0-380-76381-8

All rights reserved, which includes the right to reproduce this book or portions thereof in any form whatsoever except as provided by the U.S. Copyright Law. For information address Avon Books.

First Avon Books Trade Printing: October 1991

AVON TRADEMARK REG. U.S. PAT. OFF. AND IN OTHER COUNTRIES, MARCA REGISTRADA, HECHO EN U.S.A.

10 9 8 7 6 5 4 3 2 1

Note: Natural medicines are generally safe and effective. But, despite every effort to offer expert and well-tested advice, it is not possible for this book to predict an individual person's reactions to a particular treatment. *Always* refer to the cautions given in Part II under specific herbs, products, and therapies, before using any of the treatments recommended. If in doubt, consult a qualified doctor, physician, or practitioner of natural medicine. Neither the publisher nor the authors accept responsibility for any effects that may arise from giving or taking any type of natural medicine, or any other related remedy or form of treatment, included in this book.

Toward Light
and Love
and Power for Women

Authors
Julian Scott MA, PhD has been practising
acupuncture for more than 15 years. He
founded the Dolphin House Clinic where
many natural therapies are used. During this
time he developed an understanding of
women's energies and the difficulties that
women face in the modern world. This book
developed out of a desire to show that the
gentle yet powerful remedies of natural
medicine can help women to feel comfortable
with their womanhood, and cure complaints.
Susan Scott has been teaching the
Alexander Technique for 20 years. She has
experienced the transformation of her career-
orientated view of life into one where her
capacity as a woman is the integrating factor.
She believes that women have an enormous
capacity to be both loving and successful, but
that many women in today's world need
natural therapies to help them overcome
their difficulties, and to maintain their
positive outlook from day to day.

Specialist consultants
Robert Cran MA is Principal of the London
Centre for Yoga and Shiatsu Studies, and
practises acupuncture, Chinese herbal
medicine, Shiatsu, and Yoga therapy. He has
studied at the College of Traditional Chinese
Medicine in Nanjing. He has a special
interest in the clinical uses of Yoga methods.
**Dr Shirley Bond MB BS, LRCP, MRCS,
FFARCS** is in general practice in London.
She specializes in the treatment of women,
combining the orthodox and complementary
approaches to medicine, and is interested in
the preventative aspects of health care.
Dr Richard Donze, DO is a general practice
physician in Philadelphia, USA. He has
lectured and written widely about health
promotion through lifestyle changes and
good nutrition. An advocate of the holistic
approach, he is a regular contributor to
medical journals, television, and radio.
Frau Gisela Meyer-Wachs has been a
qualified Heilpraktiker for 25 years. After
becoming a nurse, she studied acupunture in
China, and she now works in Augsburg.

CONTENTS

Gondola

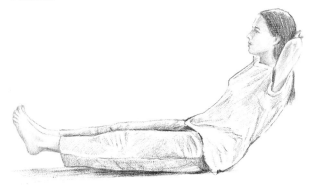

Moth

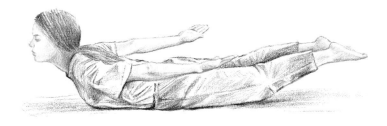

Brandysnap breathing

INTRODUCTION

We all want good health, and to enjoy life. In today's world, this means more than freeing ourselves from illness. It means living life to the full, with enhanced fitness and vitality, and a positive attitude to life. This book shows the way to better health. It aims to help you to help yourself, through understanding and using natural medicines and other natural therapies.

In recent years the belief has grown that only a professional, medically qualified physician can treat illness. This extends to minor, almost trivial ailments, so that some people feel unable to help themselves at all. This book is intended to remedy this situation. It explains how you can maintain and improve your health, by attention to diet, exercise, relationships, commitments, and other aspects of daily life. It shows how to use natural remedies in the home, for self-treatment and cure.

Whole health

Many women suffer unnecessary pain and discomfort, when an understanding of why the pain occurs, and the taking of a simple and safe natural remedy, could alleviate the problem. This extraordinary state of affairs has arisen partly because of male-dominated orthodox Western medicine. And the attitude is reinforced by our cultural traditions, in which women's problems tend to be regarded as mere frailty, and not something to discuss openly. For example, it is quite acceptable to mention that a cold in the head makes you weak and miserable. But is it as acceptable to talk freely about how period pains make you feel drained and depressed?

Fortunately, enormous changes are now taking place in our society. Old-fashioned attitudes are being replaced by more positive and open discussions of health matters. Women are rightly beginning to look for explanations, diagnosis, treatments, and cures for their illnesses and conditions.

This book is not intended to replace orthodox medicine. Rather, it aims to widen your appreciation of health, and your understanding of why you become ill. It shows that in addition to Western-style drugs and surgery, there are other, and in many cases better, treatments for health problems.

CHINESE MEDICINE

Throughout this book, there are references to various features and sayings from Chinese medicine. This bias toward the East is inevitable for authors trained in Chinese health care. However, these sayings and attitudes are not exclusively Chinese, or even Eastern, in their applications. They are Universal Truths. Their origins lie in the problems that all peoples of the world face from day to day. The cures have their foundations in the respect we should have for our own bodies and minds, and the love we feel for our partners, families, and friends.

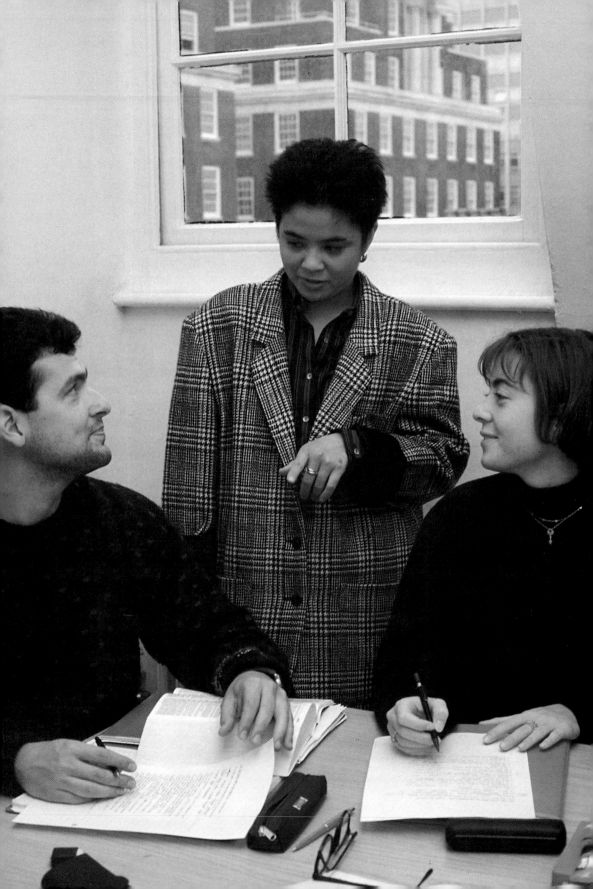

Often, natural treatments can be combined with aspects of orthodox medicine to produce a more favourable outcome. A delightful Chinese saying embodies this principle: "Walking on two legs is better than walking on one."

There are times when we want to overcome a problem on our own; at other times, we may feel unable to take on the responsibility. Certain problems are treatable at home, but others need the help of a practitioner. Do not hesitate to obtain advice if you feel you need it.

The causes of illness

One of the basic tenets of Chinese medicine is that there are always causes in life for poor health. An illness is not something that strikes mysteriously from nowhere, for no reason. It has clearly identifiable origins. Typically, the Chinese approach views the origins as an imbalance in the body, and in the body's response to an external stress.

Sometimes the external stress, such as infecting germs or an emotional upset, may be so violent that even a strong, healthy body is knocked off balance. At other times there is already an inner imbalance, and even the slightest external stress can bring on illness.

For this reason, causes of illness are an important part of this book. There are explanations of how external events can combine with the body's reactions to them, resulting in poor health. This fuller understanding brings practical benefits, in the form of effective treatments and preventing recurrence.

Disease patterns When you become ill, a varying number of minor symptoms may be associated with the main condition.

Orthodox Western medicine describes the overall picture in terms of "syndromes." In natural medicine, we refer to "patterns" of ill-health (see p.27). The patterns often cut across orthodox medicine's syndromes, seeming at times even to contradict them. Nevertheless, they are frequently seen in practice. The reason for this difference is that orthodox medicine concentrates mainly on the physical body and its symptoms, while natural medicine also takes account of the body's energy and emotions, and symptoms on the mental and spiritual levels. This wider, holistic view explains many otherwise puzzling symptoms.

How to use this book

Identifying an illness If you are worried about a health problem, and especially when using the book for the first few times, consult the Contents list or the Index. Then turn straight to the relevant pages in Part III, Treating Conditions and Ailments, where the problem that you suspect is described.

Check that your symptoms and pattern of illness correspond with those listed in the text. This should confirm your diagnosis. If something seems amiss, consult a qualified practitioner of natural or orthodox medicine for advice.

Choosing a therapy Read the general text and the various treatments advised. For each illness, there are details of three, four, or even five different therapies. These alternatives are described because some people feel more comfortable with one particular therapy. They seem to have an instinctive knowledge of how to use it. Also, some people respond well to one therapy but not to another.

Simply start with the therapy that attracts you most. Or try the remedies in the order given, or according to the contents of your medicine cupboard. As you gain experience, you may find that you react more favourably to one therapy than to the others.

Prescribing When you feel ready to prescribe a remedy, turn to the relevant pages in Part II, The Natural Therapies, for general information on the type of treatment. Read this in conjunction with any specific information for the illness, such as the dosage, and how often you should take the remedy, or how long you should do an exercise. Monitor your reactions, and take special note of any cautions or contraindications given for a particular remedy.

Finding out more about remedies You may wish to know the details of an individual remedy, such as the effects of a particular herb, or the suitability of a certain homeopathic preparation. Consult the Index and turn directly to the relevant pages in Part II, The Natural Therapies. Or scan through the Materia Medica listings in Part II to locate an individual remedy or exercise.

Background knowledge Part I, Developing Health, is a general introduction to the subject of natural medicine, with particular reference to women's problems.

Using and changing therapies In general, use only one therapy at a time. For example, select either a herbal remedy, or a homeopathic one. Do not feel that, by taking both remedies simultaneously, that you will speed their action. If one therapy does not seem to work after a few days, change to another. You can also change the therapy at different stages of the condition. For example, if you have successfully used homeopathy during the acute stage, you can switch to a herbal remedy to speed your recovery.

The exercise routines may be used in conjunction with any of the natural therapies. Indeed, it often happens that adding a specific exercise opens the way for the other remedy to work.

A note of caution: If your condition deteriorates or does not seem to be clearing, consult a qualified practitioner to confirm the diagnosis.

Taking it further

A book such as this cannot describe every illness, all fields of natural medicine, and the thousands of remedies available. If you develop a deeper interest in a specific aspect of home treatment, there are more specialized books available, as listed on p.186.

SERIOUS ILLNESS

For many of the problems described in this book, there is information on what to do should your condition become more serious. Never take chances with your health and well being. If you feel worried, for whatever reason, listen to your instincts and innermost feelings. Consult a practitioner of natural or orthodox medicine as quickly as possible.

It is far better to call in professional assistance early, and catch a potentially serious problem while it is still treatable.

Part I

DEVELOPING HEALTH

Natural medicine is concerned with life - with you as a whole person, and the way you interact with the world. Like orthodox Western medicine, it deals with the physical well being of the body, but it also takes account of the breadth of human experience: emotional, psychological, spiritual, intellectual, and sensual. It recognizes the importance of joy and sorrow, hope and regret.

Our problems and illnesses relate to experiences on different levels, not merely the physical plane. This is especially true of problems which are often classified in orthodox medicine as "functional." This term implies that nothing is actually "wrong," in the strict sense of a significant physical or physiological abnormality.

For example, most cases of menstrual pain are not symptoms of serious illness, and do not threaten life. However, the perspective of natural medicine reveals that such problems originate at other levels of existence (see p.14), thereby offering effective ways to treat and cure.

The life-force and "energy"

The body's natural tendency toward health stems from the "life-force," which is present in every one of us. The remedies in this book direct the force to enhance your vitality, thereby leading to a fuller life.

The idea of a life-force has little place in orthodox medicine, being occasionally acknowledged as a "will to live" or as part of a person's constitutional resistance to disease. But it is the key to the understanding of natural medicine. In different cultures it has various names; in this book, it is described as "energy." Although not a material substance, in the same way as water or air, this energy is nonetheless indispensable for all life. Its presence distinguishes living organisms from inanimate matter.

This concept of energy is something that we all experience in ourselves and observe in others, but it differs from the notion of "energy" in the classical sciences. Many people believe that today's science is close to describing everything that exists in the universe. In fact, it largely fails to quantify or even describe some of the most basic features of our lives - indecision and clarity, joy and sadness.

Energy and natural medicines

Energy is related to the exhilaration you feel on a bright summer morning, or the inner glow when all is going well in your life. This same energy controls and directs the physical body. When your natural flow of energy is disturbed, by problems such as blockage, stagnation, or low reserves, disease is likely to occur. Your feelings and emotions are also vitally important. A life full of joy and hope is more likely to be accompanied by good health; the opposite also tends to apply.

In any illness treated by natural medicine, the first step toward a cure is restoring your energy flow. When this happens, you should start to feel better, long before your physical body is cured.

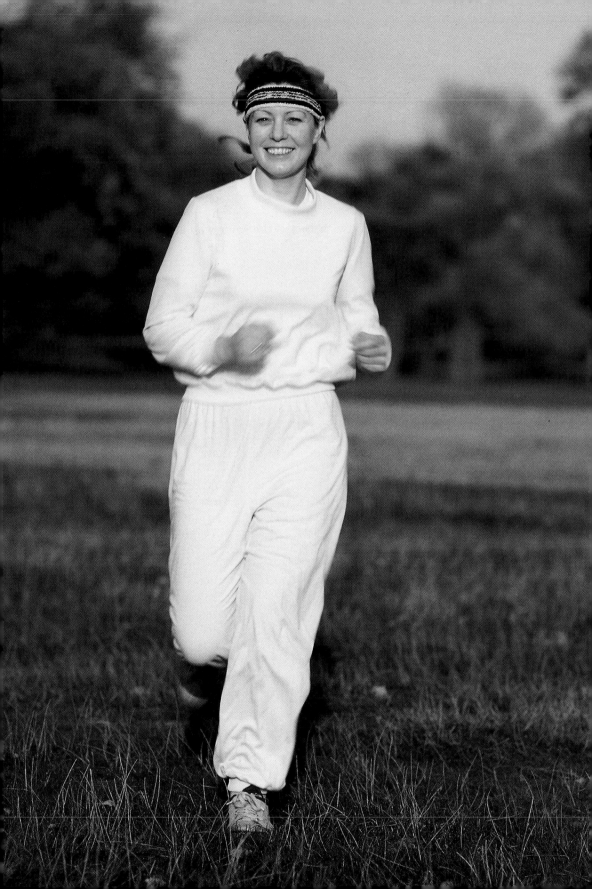

THE CONCEPT OF ENERGY

One of the most remarkable things about natural medicines is that, besides curing illnesses, they can help to increase your happiness and vitality. To understand the many actions of natural remedies, it helps to know about the various kinds of energy that make up a human being.

Classical medical philosophy, both in the West and India, describes five levels of human existence. The lowest is the physical level; above that is the vital energy level; then the emotional; then the mental; and finally the spiritual level. Each has its characteristic energy pattern, and interacts with the planes above and below.

These five levels, and the way in which a problem on one can affect the others, leading to discomfort or even disease, are central to successful treatment by natural medicines (see p.25).

Physical level

This relates to the world around us, as we see it, smell it, feel and taste and touch it. This is the level on which we are taught to understand our surroundings, through the "observable data" of science, and so it is the easiest level for most people to comprehend.

The physical level is the one we recognize as the material or "real" world, which humans have learned to dominate

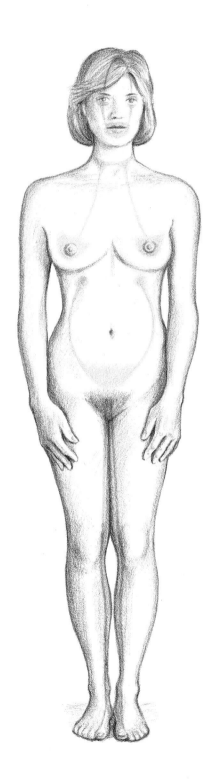

The energy channels originate in the centre of the body, from the heart, lungs, and digestive system. They radiate outward along the limbs and up into the neck and head. This representative diagram shows how the energy channels linked to the reproductive system flow toward the breasts and womb area. The channels are of great use in diagnosing and treating illness, and can be strengthened and eased by natural medicines.

with such short-term success during this century. Described by scientists and engineers, it is amenable to precise measurement and quantification. It is also the level at which orthodox medicine has had its most outstanding successes, partly because the results are so measurable.

Vital energy level

This level, although closest to the physical world, concerns the "life-force" energy that distinguishes the living from the dead or inanimate. It varies from day to day and hour to hour - sometimes you feel full of energy, at other times you have much less. After a hard day's work or a bout of influenza, your vital energy is at a low ebb. After a good vacation, it is at its peak.

This vital energy level can be enhanced by the techniques of acupuncture, healing, and massage.

Emotional level

One step from the vital energy level is the emotional level. The Buddhist religion, among others, preaches that emotions should be fleeting and soon pass, like a cloud. This concept is sometimes misunderstood, leading to the idea that emotions are not real or "useful." But most practitioners of natural medicine would refute this: while emotions should not dominate, they are as essential to higher life as vital energy.

Not only do your emotions exist, but you have a reserve of emotional energy - an "emotional body." People refer to being "emotionally drained" after watching a highly charged drama or going through a traumatic experience. In this condition, your emotional body is depleted. You lack your usual emotional energy to savour life, or even to summon up emotions such as anger or sadness.

Counselling, psychotherapeutics, and rebirthing address this level (see p.186).

Mental level

Since the advent of psychology and the behavioural sciences, most of us are familiar with the concept of the thinking mind. Thoughts and ideas are the stock-in-trade of scientists and are manipulated by the mind. Just as there are reserves of vital and emotional energy, so too there are reserves of mental power. A person can have a clear and powerful mind, without being mentally cluttered and preoccupied by thoughts.

There is a comparison between the "emotional body" and the "mental body." Just as you can be aware of your emotions, but not dominated by them, you can also be aware of your thoughts, but not obsessed by them. Like emotions, thoughts and ideas should come and go. Being stuck in a "thought rut," so that the same thought is at the forefront of your consciousness, can eventually lead to illness.

On the mental level, the techniques of homeopathy and Bach flower therapy work especially well. Also useful is positive affirmation, which has great application to allergies and problems of hypersensitivity.

Spiritual level

This level is the farthest removed from the physical. In today's materialistic world, many deny the existence of a spiritual power - though few would deny the

15

effects of a great painting or musical work. The spiritual level is the hardest for most of us to comprehend, being so far removed from the familiar physical world. Our words struggle to define it - after a momentous event, people say: "I just cannot explain my feelings." If you experience a birth or the death of a loved one, you probably recognize that the language we use for everyday matters is wholly inadequate for such fundamental, deeply-felt experiences.

Many religions and cultures teach that each of us has a "soul" or "spiritual body," which lives on after the death of the physical body. This spiritual body is the very core of human existence, the motivating force that brings life to the other levels. It is your still centre, hardly touched by the busy world. In its stillness, great ideas are born, and it is manifest to the outside world as a reserve of "creative energy" (see p.18).

Meditation, prayer, and religious ritual are especially effective in activating the spiritual body.

Being a woman

There are obvious physical and other differences between women and men. Many of the behavioural aspects have arisen through conditioning by society. As the expectations of society change, so do the relative roles of women and men. However, in Chinese philosophy, the fundamental difference is expressed in terms of energy: most women have an abundance of Yin energy, while most men possess more Yang energy.

From our Western perspective, we notice this as men being more involved with physical and vital levels, while women tend toward the emotional and

mental levels. You can observe these traits even in a child, before social conditioning and expectations have had much effect.

Such differences may arise because of a woman's capacity to bear children. During conception, pregnancy, and early infancy, the new life needs to be drawn into our world - some would say, "created from nothing." The mother supplies the spiritual, mental, emotional, and vital energy to generate this new life and nurture its early development.

As a result (and a generalization), a woman is more in touch with higher energies and levels of existence, than is a man. Her physical body may be smaller and less powerful, but her energies are directed upward to the emotional, mental, and spiritual levels.

Consequently, as a woman, you may feel that emotional and spiritual well being play an important role in health. Creating and maintaining a balance in relationships is also a significant, and often extremely demanding, part of life; and so it affects your well being. If you wish to use natural medicines, you may need to address not only your physical symptoms, but also consider these various aspects of your health and life.

Fatigue, anxiety, and the general stresses of modern life can soon deplete energy resources, especially at the emotional, mental, and spiritual levels - and often without you realizing it. In some cases this can lead to dulled mental abilities and gloomy, brooding behaviour, that does little to tackle the underlying problem. The aim is to increase your self-awareness and restore your ability to break out of repetitive, negative thought patterns. The natural remedies can assist in restoring your energy flows, so that you can tackle the problem at its root.

16

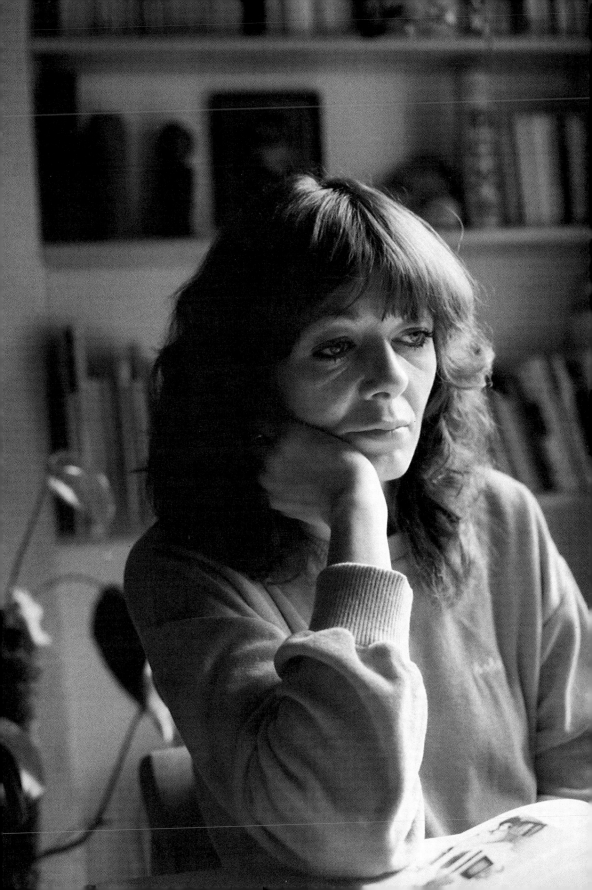

CREATIVE ENERGY

Much of the advice in this book involves the reproductive cycle, so you need to understand the views of natural medicine, and how energy moves and changes during this time.

One of the most important forms of energy is creative energy. It is closely related to your self-awareness and individuality - a still, quiet form of energy, which paradoxically causes events to happen. People with abundant creative energy inspire others to follow. They have a strong presence, a calm "power" that makes others take notice. You see this energy in great leaders in all fields - art, music, science, politics, business, and social awareness.

Creative energy nourishes your whole being. It is also the force that feeds your will, your power of thought, and your reproductive system. Knowing how this energy works can help you use it to your best advantage.

Forms of creative energy

Willpower is the strongest manifestation of creative energy. You use "will energy" to try and make something happen - for example, to guide an unwilling child, or to persuade a colleague to do a task.

Willpower energy operates when you have to get up in the middle of the night, or at any time when you must force your body to do something. However, using willpower depletes your creative energy, since it is such a concentrated form of this energy. You must then draw replacement energy from other levels.

Controlled thought is another manifestation of creative energy. When this energy is low, mental processes become slow and muddled. This can be seen in early pregnancy (when it is almost diag-nostic of the conception), and after childbirth. At such times, you may be forgetful or confused, having temporarily used up your creative energy during the pregnancy and birth.

Creative energy is, of course, involved in the creation of life. It is released during lovemaking, and provides the power for conception (see p.127).

Building up creative energy

The simplest way to build up reserves of creative energy is sleep. Your body rests, and your mind is free to wander and collect the energy for the next day.

There are two other readily-available ways of replenishing creative energy: meditation and religious worship. When you meditate (see p.70), the stillness created within your body and mind allows energy to flow in from outside, and lets you tap hitherto unrecognized sources of this energy deep within yourself. Similarly, a religious service or equivalent event brings higher forces into play, nourishing those who partake.

In general, you can strengthen your creative energy by bringing more stillness into your life, and by contacting the higher, more spiritual levels of human existence.

Depletion of creative energy

Many activities can deplete your creative energy. Two are mentioned above - willing yourself to go on when very tired, and conceiving a baby.

Creative energy is also used up during lovemaking, even if no new life is formed. Reaching orgasm brings a release of creative energy from both partners. After, they may be temporarily less inclined to get up and do things, and less able to make clear decisions. This is because the tranquility induced by orgasm diminishes their need to influence the world around. This soon passes, and if the tranquil phase is allowed to ebb naturally, sex often brings a sense of rejuvenation and renewal.

Low creative energy can affect your whole system, giving rise to a host of general symptoms, including depression, fatigue, lethargy, and exhaustion. These may extend to the physical and functional levels, affecting your reproductive organs, and leading to conditions such as pelvic floor weakness.

The power of a musical performance can affect those around, inspiring performers and listeners alike to recognize and tap their deep reserves of creative energy.

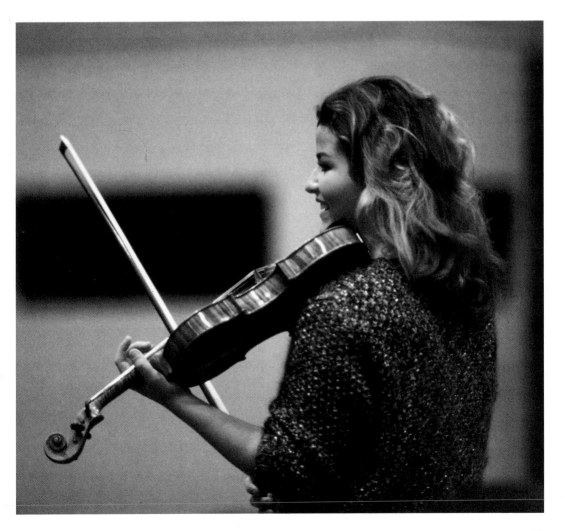

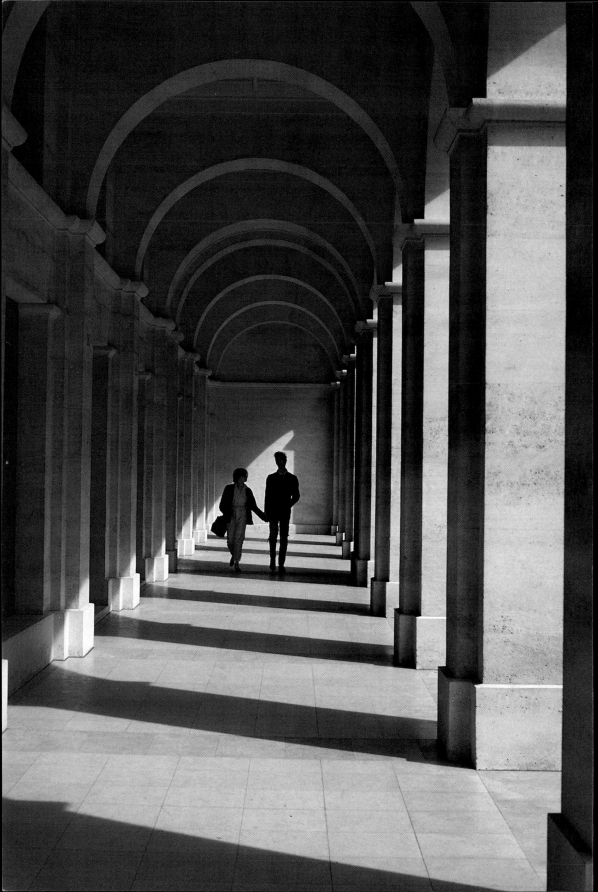

THRESHOLDS IN LIFE

The landscape in China has always been dominated by gates. Every city has a huge town wall and, until recently, the only way to enter was through a magnificent gateway. Even in the countryside, small gates represent the transition from one place to another, for example, from cultivated land to wild mountainside. What could be more natural than to describe life's important transitions or thresholds as "gates"?

In traditional societies, most women experience several main gateways in life: puberty; establishing a stable relationship (signified in many cultures by marriage or its equivalent); pregnancy and childbirth; and menopause.

At these transitions, personality and health have the opportunity to undergo great change - for better or worse. If you prepare for the transition, and take special care with your life and health at this time, a gateway can offer the chance to cure long-established illness. Even if there is no illness, provided you pay attention to yourself before and during the transition, you can enhance your well being, improve your outlook, and learn more about yourself on each level.

In contrast, if you are ill-prepared and under great stress during the transition, you run the risk of worsening health, until the next gate beckons.

Gateways today

In contemporary Western society, the gates are not so clearly defined, nor so limited, as they were in ancient China!

Gateways and arches are symbols of transition, as well as strong and stable architectural devices. Passing through them is common in Eastern and Western ceremonies.

Significant changes also occur at many other times: when a woman experiences her first sexual relationship, starts her first job, leaves home, sees her children grow up and leave home and become independent, and when she moves toward retirement.

But the changes that women experience and adapt to are still much greater than for most men. Becoming pregnant alters your whole perspective on life. You may well find that your attitudes and balance - physical, mental, and emotional - undergo radical changes.

Unfortunately, society encourages us to resist some of these changes. For example, a woman who becomes pregnant may feel resentful at her career or other aspirations being interrupted. This is not because of the interruption itself, but because many professions (especially male-dominated ones) take little account of, or even disapprove of, this phase in a woman's life.

Puberty

At puberty, individuality becomes more strongly defined. This is the time when your creative energy (see p.18) comes into play, as reflected on the physical level by the start of menstruation.

It is very important to keep the energy flowing by physical activity, and to avoid exhaustion, particularly from too much schoolwork. Menstrual problems, even in later life, may sometimes be traced back to stress from schoolwork during puberty. Or they may be rooted in fearful notions instilled by well-meaning parents, friends, or relatives, that periods are supposed to be painful and unpleasant, and you have to suffer. This is not so. If there are problems when

21

HELPFUL REMEDIES FOR PUBERTY

As puberty approaches, girls commonly have difficulty controlling negative emotions. The best way to help is by the old remedy of "tender loving care." On the physical level, they usually have problems of mucus accumulation, including chronic coughs, oily skin, and nasal congestion. The following herbal remedies should help, and also assist relaxation and developing personality.

- Golden seal (*Hydrastis canadensis*).
- Elecampane (*Inula helenium*).
- Hyssop (*Hyssopus officinale*).
- Coltsfoot (*Tussilago farfara*).

Mix equal quantities of each herb, and take 20-30 drops of the mixture in water, 3 times daily.
- Or take a cupful of tea made from one teaspoon of Heartsease (*Viola tricolor*), 3 times daily.
- Skin rashes are also common at this time, especially for the girl who has not had measles, since puberty is an opportunity to throw out poisons which should have been expelled from the body during childhood. A daily cup of tea made from Yarrow (*Achillea millefolium*) for several months can also help to cure skin rashes.

periods start, consult a practitioner of natural medicine. During this time, avoid mucus-producing foods such as milk, cheese, and peanuts (see p.31). Eat red meat sparingly.

Marriage or its equivalent

In the past, marriage was a much greater transition than it is for most of us in the West today. A woman left her home and perhaps her town or village, and became part of a new, extended family, often under the rule of her new parents-in-law.

In the West, there are many different versions of this transition. You may undergo a more gradual change, from being unattached and living with parents, then dating, to eventually establishing a firm relationship with a partner, and perhaps living together before marriage - if this ever occurs.

This sequence of events, without clear transitions, does not present the same

opportunity for changes in health. However, there is still a strong opportunity - at marriage itself, which usually marks a definite and deeper step than the decision to live together. It is the very depth of this decision that can provide you with the gateway to enhanced health.

Childbirth

Giving birth, especially to your first child, is a time when your health can take a great turn for the better - or worse. After giving birth, you may well feel a sense of completion, fulfillment, and new confidence. For the first time in your life, you have a courage and determination that you never thought possible, particularly concerning your baby.

You may also experience these changes on the physical level, in the form of greater energy and stamina. Equally, it is a time when many period problems that started at puberty can finally disappear. If the birth goes badly, though, the resulting weakness and exhaustion are very difficult to overcome. Some women even remark that their health and energy after birth never really returned to previous levels, but stayed low for years. Natural medicines can help to restore energy and well being, and give a more positive outlook.

Preparation for childbirth The main preparation is rest. Spend an hour relaxing some time during the day. If you work, try to rearrange your hours or have a longer midday break. If you have other children, ask your partner or someone else to look after them, so that you still get your rest. Eat healthy food, avoid tobacco and alcohol, get regular and gentle exercise, and generally take things more slowly.

During your pregnancy, particularly in the last three months, take Raspberry leaf (*Rubus idaeus*) as tea or tablets, to tone the uterine muscles. Another herb with the same effect is Beth root (*Trillium pendulum*), also known as Birth root, taken during the last month as an alternative to Raspberry leaf. Remedies that can ease childbirth are listed on p.147.

After childbirth Giving birth can be a wonderful experience, but exhausting on several levels. If you are excessively tired, or you experienced a traumatic labour, consult a practitioner of natural medicine.

During pregnancy, try to find enough time and an appropriately serene place, to rest and conserve energy. This is one of the most important aspects of preparing for the birth.

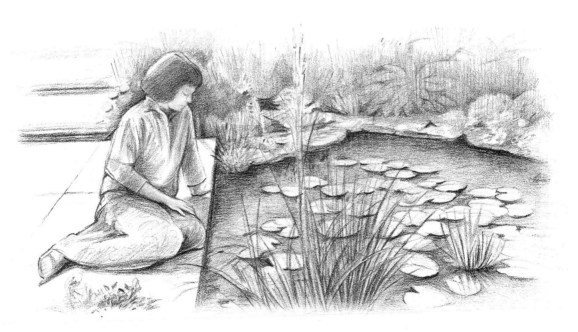

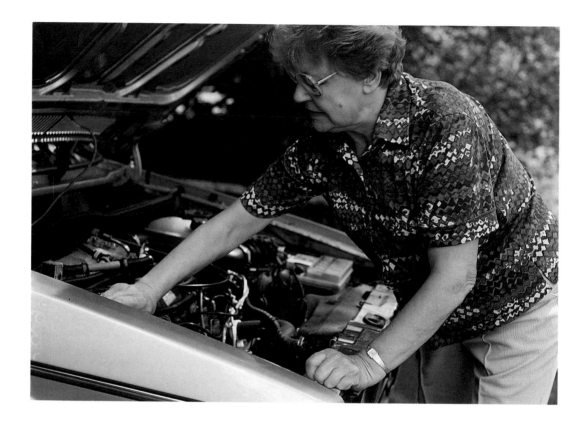

The menopause is a fine opportunity for making a "fresh start." Consider an activity that you truly want to do, rather than something which you feel you ought to be pursuing.

Menopause

This presents another chance to change your health. For example, if you have experienced painful or otherwise troublesome periods, this is the time when they stop. However, if you are overstretched during this transition, you may suffer from postmenopausal problems. Take care of your health during this transition, and you have the opportunity to improve your constitution, and enjoy a fulfilled "third age."

Retirement

When you work, and/or look after a partner, and/or a family, you have a reason for getting up and starting the day. People depend on you and appreciate your efforts (even though the appreciation may come in the form of a regular paycheque).

At retirement, this usually changes, and you may need to find new outlets for your continuing creative energy. Often this is no problem, but if you have a demanding job, it can be difficult to establish a new pattern. You may have problems linked to unbalanced, blocked, or weak energy. Consult a practitioner, as well as trying natural medicines.

ENERGY IMBALANCES

When you are healthy, energy flows strongly and vigorously throughout your body, enabling it to function well. However, the energy can sometimes become blocked, so that it fails to reach the areas where it is needed. This can lead to illness.

Energy blocks

For example, anxiety and worry may block energy flow from the stomach, so that it cannot spread down to the intestines. The result may be heaviness and pain in the stomach, where the energy is blocked, and also diarrhoea, since the intestines lack enough energy to complete their digestion of food.

Energy blocks can occur anywhere in the body. In the limbs, they cause symptoms such as cramps, weakness, or tingling; in the internal organs, they lead to conditions such as irregular or difficult periods (see p.120).

Energy shortages

Women often experience a shortage of total energy. This is especially common when you are tired or exhausted, particularly after a long illness, after childbirth, when looking after children single-handed, or if you have both a family and a career. Energy shortage may lead to the "energy exhaustion pattern" (see p.28) and the associated "weak" patterns of certain illnesses, for example, anaemia (see p.93).

Energy imbalance and emotions

Emotions play an important part in directing the flow of energy. Positive emotions of happiness, joy, and enthusiasm tend to increase the quantity and flow of energy (which is why we call them "positive"). They produce balanced and uniform patterns of energy distribution, that can sustain your body in health for prolonged periods of time.

Negative emotions such as depression, apathy, and fear tend to decrease the amount of energy. They produce rather unbalanced or blocked patterns of flow that, if prolonged, may open the way for disquiet and disease.

As explained on p.12, many of the problems discussed in this book are referred to in orthodox Western medicine as "functional" disorders. The perspective of natural medicine reveals that they are not really centred on the physical level, but originate from higher aspects of your being, most often the vital energy and emotional levels (see p.15).

The emotional level controls vital energy. Therefore even a small emotional imbalance can significantly upset your vital energy. This is why natural medicine emphasizes the emotional factors in illness, since these often provide the clues to the correct advice and treatment.

Energy interactions

Once you understand the perspective of natural medicine, and the ways in which your five different energy levels interact, you can see how imbalance at any level may cause fatigue, depression, or illness. Initially, the malaise is confined to one level; but if the imbalance persists, it is likely to spread.

For example, if you feel insecure in your work, a common reaction is worry. In the early stages, this develops into anxiety, but the problem is usually confined to the emotional level. Doing something pleasurable is often sufficient to disperse the anxiety temporarily. However, if it continues, it begins to affect your vital energy level. Commonly this manifests itself as an energy blockage in the upper abdomen (see diagram), which you feel as a slight weight in the stomach and minor indigestion.

If the problem persists, the blockage of vital energy can become more severe, leading to bad pains from indigestion, stomach cramps, and vomiting. These are signs of an incipient stomach ulcer.

The blockage may remain at the vital energy level, without spreading to the physical level. Should the energy block remain, your physical body might eventually be affected by an actual ulcer.

Diagnosis and treatment

This example of the stomach ulcer illustrates how the levels of existence interact, and how an energy imbalance can spread to cause discomfort, pain, malaise, and even physical illness.

It is well known in orthodox medicine that stomach ulcers are linked to worry, stress, and anxiety. But in natural medicine, it is believed that almost any illness involves energy imbalances, not only on the physical level but on other planes, too. Indeed, most illnesses are said to originate from emotional, mental, and spiritual components, rather than physical ones. The skill in diagnosis lies

in determining the level on which the problem emanates, and selecting treatments which benefit that level.

Sometimes you may find it sufficient to treat an illness solely on the physical level. More often, however, you need to attend to your emotional or vital energy levels for success. With a serious disease such as cancer, treatment is needed on every level, from the physical through to the spiritual.

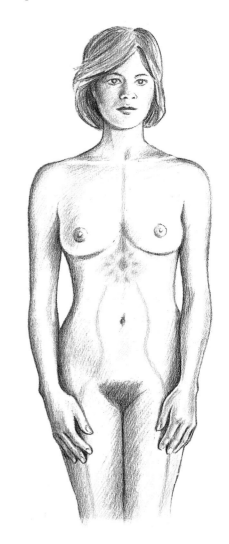

This diagrammatic representation shows the disrupted energy pattern linked to stomach ulcer. It reveals stagnation down the stomach channel, where stiffness may be felt. Treatment involving this channel can relieve the blockage, thereby initiating a cure.

PATTERNS OF ILL HEALTH

If you become ill, it is likely that you have not one symptom, but a collection of related symptoms. Orthodox medicine refers to these characteristic symptom groups as "syndromes." Each syndrome is viewed as a collection of physical manifestations that originate from connected problems in the physical body. Treatment is usually symptomatic: it focuses on the major symptoms, and does not necessarily strike at the cause.

The significance of disease patterns

In natural medicine, a characteristic group of symptoms is called a "pattern." The pattern is often more significant than the main symptom, since it is the pattern that determines correct treatment. This is because it points to the cause, thereby offering the solution. With the perspective of natural medicine, you can often identify the simple imbalance that provides the connecting link between the symptoms. This helps to make the overall pattern of the illness intelligible.

Patterns are also important because many of them relate to the level at which the imbalance or blockage lies. If you have an illness stemming from a problem on the emotional level (such as prolonged frustration), this will have a quite different pattern from an illness originating at the vital energy level (such as prolonged overwork or sleeplessness). Each of these patterns requires you to use different remedies and apply different changes to your lifestyle.

The major "hot" and "cold" patterns described below are very common. They are related to everyday experience, when you might feel either too warm and flushed after great activity or hot weather, or shivery and chilled in an unexpected cold wind.

Two other common patterns described here are "poor energy circulation" and "energy exhaustion." In traditional Chinese medicine, the main internal organ concerned with energy circulation is the liver, and many of the symptoms listed for these patterns are related to the liver and its functions.

"Hot" and "cold" patterns

The "hot" pattern is one of the most common types of ill-health. If you suffer from a "hot" illness, you develop signs of

HOT AND COLD PATTERNS	
Hot	*Cold*
Red face	White face
Tendency to inflammation and burning pains	Tendency to cramping pains
Liking for cool weather	Liking for warm weather
Preference for thin, light clothes	Preference for thick clothes
Liking for cool foods and cold-energy foods (see p.32)	Liking for warm foods and hot-energy foods (see p.33)

the illness itself, but these are biased toward the types of symptoms that occur when your body gets too hot, or when you are in warm surroundings, or indications of heat and inflammation throughout your body.

For example, if you have a "hot"-type stomach disorder, you probably feel burning sensations in your stomach, and you react poorly to hot weather, hot foods, and hot drinks. You may have bodily signs of heat and inflammation, such as a flushed face, sore and red eyes, and a harsh and swollen throat. You may find yourself counteracting the increased heat by wearing light clothes, compared to other people.

The "cold" patterns of illness involve signs you may develop when your body becomes chilled, such as a pale face, shivering, and cramping pains in the limbs or lower abdomen.

"Poor energy circulation" pattern

If you suffer from an illness of this pattern, your symptoms are likely to be related to irritability and anger. When a

POOR ENERGY CIRCULATION PATTERN

Irritability before a period
Sore breasts
Cold hands and feet
Hot sensations inside
Preference for vegetables over meat
Feeling worse after drinking coffee
Feeling better after exercise, and after alcohol, but a tendency to hangover headaches

problem crops up, you may become angry and fly into a rage. Conversely, if you experience prolonged anger and resentment, you may develop an illness involving poor energy circulation. Moving foods (see p.31) can be helpful in combatting this type of ill health.

"Energy exhaustion" pattern

This problem develops when your body's supply of energy is used up. It can occur

ENERGY EXHAUSTION PATTERN

Sore, weak back
Tendency to muscular weakness, for example, in the pelvic floor or bladder (see p.155)
Tendency to anaemia
Feeling worse after exercise
Poor appetite, or never satisfied after a meal

from lack of sleep or prolonged overwork, or after giving birth. Its causes are described in detail elsewhere (see, for example, p.106), and several of the strengthening (tonic) foods that counteract it are listed on p.30.

A HEALTHY DIET

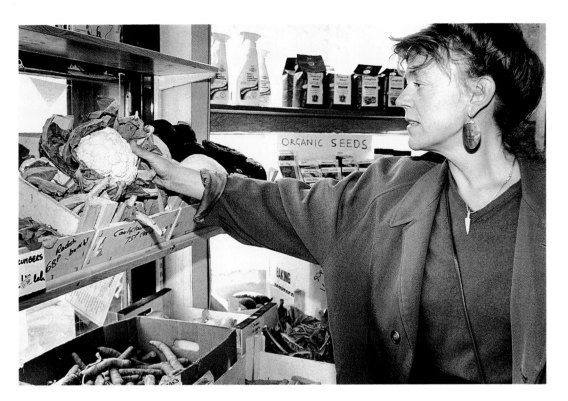

Diet plays a crucial part in health. Controversy has always surrounded the subject, with vigorous and continuing debates on every aspect of nutrition. Arguments about the merits of white bread versus brown go back to classical Greek times. Early writings on medicine, ascribed to Hippocrates in Greece and the Yellow Emperor of China, have extensive sections on diet.

Although not the main subject of this book, diet is a vital element in the healing approach of natural medicine. For many ailments, there is advice on therapeutic foods and drinks to speed your recovery, and the following pages outline the chief principles in the "natural" approach to food. This information should help to increase awareness of food's effects on your body.

Choose food for the quality of its energy rather than solely for appearance. Organically grown food sometimes shows a blemished appearance, but its vitality and flavour are usually greater, and it contains the various minerals needed for a healthy body.

Food and energy

The key principle relating diet to natural medicine is energy (see p.14). There are more aspects to a living being than the physical component. Therefore, while the physical properties of foods are important (vitamins, minerals, proteins, carbohydrates, and so on), even more vital are the energies they contain.

This may sound strange, but it is probably something you instinctively know. To understand the energy in food, think of the difference between freshly picked lettuce from the garden, and lettuce that has languished for days on a shelf. You might talk of energy and foods in the same way, calling a lettuce "tired" or "weak." Although tired lettuce has nearly the same nutrients as fresh lettuce, you instinctively feel that the latter is better. The fresh garden lettuce has the vitality essential for good health.

Organic food

The debate comparing organically grown food with food grown with artificial fertilizers concentrates on physical factors, such as the absence of trace elements, or the presence of pesticides. Yet equally important is the vital energy of your food. For example, a vegetable grown with artificial fertilizer is often larger than one grown without (that is why fertilizer is used). But its energy is less, because its vitality has been used up in rapid physical growth. So while the artificial-fertilizer-grown specimen may look impressive, it will have little natural energy and be watery, lifeless, and probably tasteless.

Heating and cooling foods

The nature of the vitality in your food is just as important as its overall energy. Just as there are "hot" and "cold" patterns in illness (see p.27), so some foods generate heat in the body, while others reduce it.

We instinctively choose heating foods in winter - stews, rich foods, soups, and broths. Cooling foods are appropriate for a hot summer's day - salads, raw foods, and fruit. The table on pp.32-33 lists the different effects of various foods.

Strengthening foods

Sometimes called "tonics," strengthening foods are particularly helpful if you suffer from energy lack or weakness, such as the "energy exhaustion" pattern of illness (see p.28). You may experience such signs in a mild form after lengthy exercise, such as after a 20-mile walk, and in a more severe form after illness or childbirth.

This weakness is not always the same as feeling tired; the latter can occur when you possess energy but its circulation has become slow or blocked, as in the "poor energy circulation" pattern (see p.28). In both cases you feel fatigued and heavy. But the weakness or lack usually stems from genuine energy exhaustion, and responds to strengthening foods. Poor energy circulation, from general inactivity, responds to moving foods (opposite).

Strengthening foods supply you with energy, but this is only useful if it circulates. So combine strengthening foods

---

STRENGTHENING FOODS

Strong tonics
All red meats; game, especially pigeon, pheasant; tuna fish
Dark meat of free-range chicken
Chocolate, cocoa
Tofu (bean curd)
Eggs

Mild tonics
White meats such as rabbit, white meat of chicken; most fish
Most nuts, such as chestnuts
Yams

with moving ones. A brief look at the two food categories shows that such a strategy is common sense. It also illustrates a general principle of natural medicine - always combine strengthening (tonic) foods and remedies with moving foods. Strengtheners on their own slow energy circulation further, leading to stagnation and blockage. This is a problem in our society, because strengthening foods and medicines are readily available, without the balance of moving foods.

Moving and stagnating foods

Moving foods encourage the movement and circulation of energy in your body. You should combine them with strengthening foods; the balance is important. As machines take over the drudgery of hard physical labour, most of us no longer need plenty of strengthening foods, which provide large amounts of energy. We have an increasing need for moving foods, which circulate and spread the energy. If you have a sedentary lifestyle, too much energy without enough circulation may cause problems. Consider a radical change of food for a trial period. Switch to a diet consisting mainly of raw foods such as vegetables (see below).

The opposites of moving foods are stagnating ones. They include strengthening foods and those called "liverish."

Side-effects If your energy reserves are very depleted, you may find that too many moving foods, without a balance of strengthening foods, can undermine your health. As a guiding principle, most people benefit from eating a diet of raw foods, such as vegetables and fruits, for about two weeks. If you plan to continue for longer, consult a dietary expert.

MOVING AND STAGNATING FOODS

Moving foods
Vegetables and fruits, especially raw
Bran and wholemeal foods such as brown rice, wholegrain brown bread

Stagnating foods
All strengthening foods (opposite)
Potatoes
Sugar, chocolate
Coffee
Fatty foods (cream, butter, fats, oils)

Protein and iron deficiencies may result from a diet containing incorrect quantities and variety of raw vegetables.

Mucus-producing and reducing foods

Another major category concerns foods that tend to increase mucus (phlegm or catarrh) in your body. This aspect of food

---

FOODS THAT AFFECT MUCUS

Mucus-forming foods
Strengthening foods (opposite)
Milk, cheese
Banana or orange (in excess)
Peanuts
Greasy foods
Alcohol or breads, in some people

Mucus-reducing foods
Moving foods (above)
Onion, garlic
Watercress
Mustard, horseradish

COLD FOODS

Apple Reduce the cool effect by cooking with cloves; raw apple may cause digestive and menstrual cramps

Banana Very cold; can relieve constipation; too much causes mucus

Celery

Cottage cheese

Cucumber Very cold

Grapefruit

Lettuce A rather "windy" or "gassy" food

Squash (vegetable marrow) Helps to reduce heating effect of lamb

Melon Reduce the cool effect by serving with ginger

Mussels Avoid if prone to allergies or rashes

Pear Reduce the cool effect by cooking with cloves; raw pears help sore throats

Yogurt Very cold; reduces the heating effects of spices

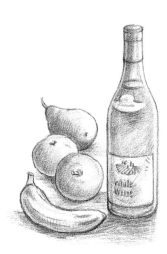

COOL FOODS

Aubergine (egg plant)

Barley Barley water is refreshing in fevers

Calf's liver Helpful for anaemia; but avoid too much in pregnancy, since it contains large amounts of vitamin A

Cow's milk Counteract the cool nature by simmering with an onion, which makes it taste sweet and reduces its mucus-forming activity

Crab Avoid during pregnancy and breastfeeding

Cress Helps to disperse phlegm

Egg plant (aubergine)

Green lentils

Lamb's liver See calf's liver

Lemon Honey and lemon juice is a refreshing drink in fevers

Mung beans

Pork Cook in soy sauce and ginger to reduce its cold nature

Soft cheeses Reduce the heat of red wine

Soused herring

Soy (soya) milk A valuable substitute for cow's milk

Spinach See p.93

Tea Green tea is a diuretic and also helps to rid the metabolism of fat, and so is a dieting aid

Tofu (bean curd) High in protein and calcium

Tomatoes (raw)

White wine Bad for arthritis

NEUTRAL FOODS

Broad beans The skins are the "gassy" part

Rice

Coconut

Corn (maize) High in phytic acid, which makes the iron difficult to absorb; neutralize by eating with chilli peppers

Dates Helpful in anaemia

Eggs Hard-boiled eggs are often difficult to digest and constipating

Grapes Strengthening in anaemia

Herring

Mushrooms Mildly active against energy blockages

Peas

Potatoes A "wet" food; overconsumption can lead to congestion and heaviness; reduce the "wet" nature by baking

Plums

Runner (string) beans

Strawberries Can cause an allergic reaction

Veal

Wheat See p.34

White cabbage

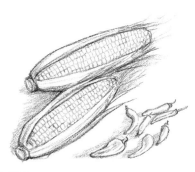

WARM FOODS

Blackberries (cooked)
Carrots
Chocolate Strengthening in cold, damp weather, but overconsumption easily leads to mucus and liverishness; may be a migraine "trigger" factor (see p.176)
Chicken Strengthening, especially after childbirth
Cocoa Same as chocolate
Coffee Helps concentration; useful in sunstroke; may worsen period pains and migraine
Figs Help relieve constipation
Goat's milk Better than cow's milk if there is a tendency to produce mucus; counteract the high sodium content by serving with celery
Greens (brassicas)
Indian tea Overconsumption can lead to stomach problems, intestinal cramps and sore back
Mint tea Promotes perspiration in fevers
Oats Strengthens the nervous system, helps to stabilize the sugar balance
Onions Help to reduce phlegm; overconsumption can increase the need for sleep
Orange Avoid in pregnancy (see p.128); the peel of bitter oranges (as in marmalade) can reduce mucus; avoid if at risk of migraine

Parsnips
Peanuts Roast peanuts can cause a lot of mucus, so avoid in chronic cough or eczema; can also cause an allergic rash
Pig's liver
Pumpkin
Radish Helps to reduce mucus
Red beans Poisonous if undercooked; tend to cause wind (gas) when cooked, so always cook with cloves
Red wine May be a "trigger" factor in migraine and arthritis
Sesame seeds High in calcium
Tomatoes (cooked)
Turnips Tend to cause wind (gas); more digestible if seasoned with nutmeg; help to promote milk flow when breastfeeding
Venison

HOT FOODS

Almonds Bitter almonds are good for the lungs
Beet (including beetroot)
Brown lentils
Brussel sprouts
Cayenne pepper Helps to expel intestinal worms
Cinnamon Add to tea to promote perspiration in colds; can cause heart palpitations and insomnia
Cloves Especially useful for dispersing flatulence and stomach discomfort; add to all bean dishes to promote digestibility
Eels
Garlic Reduces mucus and prevents colds; overconsumption can lead to sore, red eyes; avoid in psoriasis
Ginger Strengthens a weak digestion; too much can burn the stomach
Lamb
Peaches
Pepper (black)

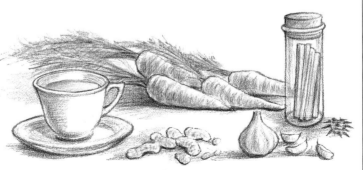

has not yet been adequately researched in orthodox medicine. In natural medicine, the effects of these foods depend on your digestive constitution. A strong digestion should be able to cope with most foods, without producing excess mucus. Energy stagnation, or too many mucus-forming foods, can result in excess mucus (see, for example, p.102).

Some people find that foods made with yeast (for example, bread or beer) tend to cause excess mucus.

Gluten

Some people cannot cope with gluten (a wheat protein) in food. Gluten is contained in wheat and wheat products such as bread, pastas, and biscuits. In extreme cases it causes the orthodox medical syndrome of coeliac disease. In mild cases, which often pass unrecognized, the main features are an increase in mucus and a general sense of heaviness and lethargy. If you feel you may be sensitive to gluten, consult a practitioner of natural or orthodox medicine.

Food combining

If you have a weak digestion, you can obtain more strength and nourishment from food by eating mainly proteins, or chiefly carbohydrates, at each meal. This means sorting foods into those that contain predominantly carbohydrate, and those that are mostly protein, and taking them at separate meals.

Research shows that these two types of foods are best digested at different acidity levels in the stomach, and that you respond to each type of food by producing the necessary amounts of acids and digestive enzymes. So improve your digestion, and extract the maximum nutrition from your foods, by keeping proteins and carbohydrates largely separate. This is known as "food combining" or the "Hay method" (see p.186).

To be a vegetarian?

Attitudes to food vary enormously, as does the supply of food in different countries. You may feel that all food is to be enjoyed; or you may have religious beliefs, or a concern for animal welfare, that prevents you eating meat - or at least, some forms of it.

Why should we eat meat? There are good nutritional and medical reasons. It is a great tonic if you are weak or debilitated. Dietetic advice may recommend a meat-containing diet if you become anaemic. Some forms of anaemia, particularly during pregnancy and/or periods of overwork, are so severe that a vegetarian diet will not relieve the problem.

Arguments against meat are also very forceful. If you consume it, you are taking the life of another living creature, however indirectly. In Western society, livestock animals are often reared in inhumane conditions and fed an unnatural diet; when eating meat, you absorb any poisons in their food, and also the bad energy created by their miserable living conditions.

From the medical point of view, there are arguments against meat. It is too rich for most Westerners, with their sedentary life style. Overconsumption can make you physically heavy, and rather dull and unresponsive on the emotional and spiritual planes, so that you are preoccupied with the material world and possessions, at the expense of spiritual fulfillment.

This ability of excess meat to change the balance of energy, from the spiritual toward the physical, is reflected by many religions, some of which proscribe meat at certain times. The striking fact emerges that great religions see meat as a barrier to spiritual development.

Striking a balance There is a reverse side, because there may be times when you become slightly too removed from the physical world. The balance topples the other way, so that you may be spiritually content, yet weak and ineffective when interacting with the physical world. This is especially common during and just after pregnancy, and after illness. In pregnancy and birth, the main focus is bringing a new soul into the world, with emphasis on creating a physical body for it. If you are not sufficiently materially orientated and "grounded," the baby may be affected. This does not mean you must eat meat in pregnancy - only that, for some women, meat can help to create a secure physical foundation for the new child. Likewise, meat can speed a return to health after severe illness.

Good-quality vegetarian food can fulfill the body's energy and nutrient needs, provided the ingredients are correctly balanced.

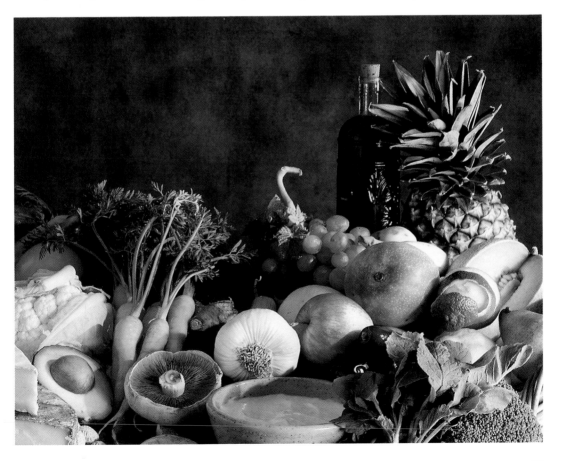

Part II

THE NATURAL THERAPIES

Natural therapies have been used for centuries. However, in recent times, people in the West have largely lost sight of nature's cures, due to the rise in orthodox medicine, and its preoccupation (in some regions) with physical symptoms, batteries of synthetic drugs, and an increasing reliance on technical tests and surgery.

The natural therapies outlined in the following pages represent a generally simple, safe, and effective approach, especially to most of the common and less serious ailments which affect women. As you begin to prescribe and use natural medicines, you will become more aware of your condition - not only in your physical body, but also on your emotional, mental, and spiritual levels. You will be able to recognize the therapies with which you feel most at ease, and identify which are most effective for your own constitution.

CAUTIONS

In general, herbal and homeopathic remedies and exercise routines are safe at all times. Some should be restricted in certain situations, such as pregnancy or during your period, as indicated in the Materia Medica.

Always check that the remedy you wish to use is suitable for your condition and for your particular case. If there is any doubt, or if you do not have the details of a remedy at hand, do not use it. Consult a qualified practitioner of natural medicine for further advice.

Organization and use

This part of the book contains details of many dozens of herbal preparations, homeopathic remedies, and therapeutic exercise positions and routines. The introductory pages to each of these therapies provide you with basic, practical background knowledge.

The herbs and homeopathic remedies are listed alphabetically by their internationally recognized names (the scientific Latin or botanical names in the case of herbs).

The exercises are graded from the less demanding Weak and Easy Stretch "beginner's routines" to the more strenuous Strong and Dynamic routines. In addition, various single-posture exercises are described in detail in Part III of the book, under the condition for which they are most beneficial.

This part of the book may be used in two ways. First, you can regard it as a back-up to the third part, Treating Conditions and Ailments, as explained on pp.10-11.

Second, the Materia Medica listings will help you prescribe your own remedies. For example, you may develop a condition not described in Part III. Or you may find that a particular herb or other remedy is strikingly effective when you use it, and you wish to know more about its wider application. In such cases, refer directly to the following pages, where the remedy should be described in detail.

For remedies not included here, consult the list of more specialized publications on p.186.

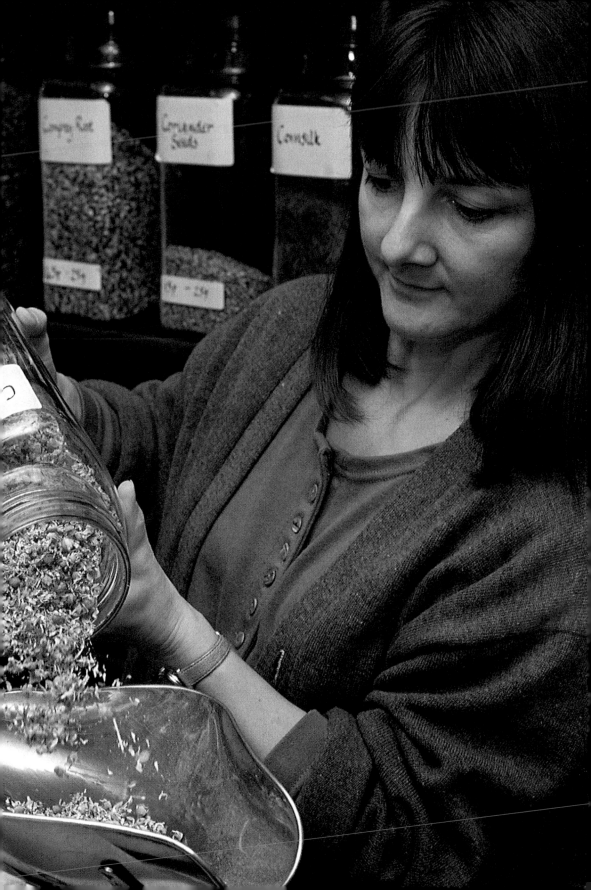

HERBAL MEDICINE

Herbs and other plants have been used for healing since the earliest times, in all civilizations and cultures. About half of the drugs in modern Western medicine were first derived from plants.

Herbal medicine works on many levels. The most obvious is the physical effect, when a relatively large amount of the remedy is consumed. In quantity, some herbs nourish in much the same way as foods. More recently, people have begun to use herbs medicinally, in much smaller amounts - and they are just as effective. This is because even quite small quantities of a properly prepared plant extract contain the life-force - the energy or "vibration" (see p.12) - of the plant itself. Remedies are prepared to retain much of the plant's energy, which increases and directs your own energy.

In contrast, Western orthodox medicine tends to focus on the body's physical symptoms. Its remedies are prepared by technical processes such as sterilization and chemical synthesis, which destroy any life-force and energy, leaving only the material substance.

Herbal medicine works on an energetic level, which particularly recommends it for menstrual problems (see p.88). The remedies act to dissolve energy blocks and straighten kinks in energy pathways, thereby helping the body's natural self-healing powers.

Obtaining herbs

Dried herbs and the various preparations made from them, such as tinctures, are readily available from most health food stores, pharmacies, and other commercial suppliers (see p.187). If you are unable to locate a source, a local herbalist or practitioner of natural medicine should be able to help. Ready-to-use herbal preparations are convenient, save wastage, usually taste pleasant, and are rarely expensive.

If you wish to dry and prepare your own remedies, many of the herbs mentioned here can be grown in gardens or found in the wild. Garden suppliers and seed merchants usually have a selection of medicinal herbs, often by mailorder. If you gather herbs from the wild, bear in mind the following points:

● Observe wildlife laws and obtain the landowner's permission to take plants.

● Enlist the help of a knowledgeable person, to be absolutely sure that you have identified the herb correctly.

● Pick only fresh and healthy plants, untouched by pesticides and other chemicals, and as clean as you would expect your food to be.

Types of herbal preparations

Information on preparation of individual herbs, such as which part(s) of the plant you should use, is given on pp.42-53.

Infusion (tea) Make an infusion by pouring hot (usually boiling) water over the relevant part of the herb. In effect, it is a herb tea. This is the preferred method for herbs containing volatile oils, which are the main substances that give the aroma, taste, and medicinal value, and which the hot water dissolves out of the herb.

To make a standard infusion, add one heaped 5mls teaspoon of dried herb to a regular teacup (about 250mls or 8fl ozs) of hot water. Stir in the herb, leave it for a few minutes, then strain off the solids to leave the liquid infusion, which you can drink as it cools. Some herbs, such as Chamomile, are available as tea-bags.

The infusion method is unsuitable for preparing root extracts, since roots take longer to release their constituents.

Decoction This is made by simmering the dried herb in water for 10-30 minutes, in a non-metallic pan (non-stick, enamel, or glass). Use three heaped 5mls teaspoonfuls of the powdered herb to 500mls (about one pint) of water. The solids are strained off to obtain the liquid decoction. This method is best for roots and a few herbs with less soluble compounds.

Tincture Prepare this extract by macerating (soaking) the dried, powdered herb in an alcohol/water mixture. Most tinctures are prepared at 1:5, that is, 1 part of herb to 5 parts of alcohol/water mixture. This is the "mother tincture." The alcohol preserves and stabilizes the extract.

To make the alcohol/water mixture, add one volume of alcohol to three times that volume of water, and stir well. The recommended form of alcohol is medicinal quality ethyl alcohol. This may be available from pharmacies or similar suppliers, or from herbalists. If not, it is possible to use a spirit such as brandy.

It takes about one week to prepare a tincture from leaves, and three weeks or more for roots.

Standard dosages

If there are no specific instructions for dosages in the following pages, or under the ailment in question in Part III, follow these guidelines.

For dried herbs, the standard adult dose is one heaped 5mls teaspoon of powdered leaves, or one level 5mls teaspoon of powdered roots. The herbs may be taken dry and washed down with water,

or drunk as an infusion or decoction. Girls under about 15 years of age should take half the adult dose. Unless directed, take one dose three times daily for chronic conditions, and one dose every two or three hours for acute conditions.

For an infusion or decoction, prepare the herb as described above. Drink the equivalent of a regular teacup of infusion, or one wineglassful (about 100mls or 2fl ozs) of decoction, three times daily.

For a tincture, the standard adult dose is 10 drops of mother tincture of each herb, three times daily. Use an approved medical-type dropper bottle to measure the drops. This gives a single drop volume of about 0.04mls (25 drops per millilitre). *Caution:* Always take tinctures in water, never neat (undiluted). Add them to water or a dilute drink, and sip this slowly. The alcohol in undiluted tinctures can burn the mouth.

DOSES AND REACTIONS

Typical doses of herbs today are far smaller than in the past, because we recognize that much of the healing effect depends on the plant's energy. This means the exact amount of herb is less important, compared to the dosages for orthodox medical drugs.

Provided you follow the instructions and observe the cautions for each remedy, the herbs and dose levels in this book should be safe. However, a few people are especially sensitive or allergic to a particular herb. If you develop any unusual reactions after taking a remedy, stop the treatment and contact a practitioner of natural medicine for advice.

INDEX OF HERBS	Page	Common name	Scientific name
Herbs in the Materia Medica (see pp.42-53) are listed in alphabetical order using their international scientific (Latin) names. The index on the right enables you to locate an individual herb using its common, everyday name. The scientific and common names of all remedies are also listed in the main Index (see p.188)	46	American cranesbill	*Geranium maculatum*
		American valerian	see **Lady's slipper**
	52	Beth root	*Trillium pendulum*
		Birth root	see **Beth root**
	44	Black cohosh	*Cimicifuga racemosa*
	48	Black root	*Leptandra virginica*
	43	Blue cohosh	*Caulophyllum thalactroides*
		Bottlebrush	see **Horsetails**
		Buckthorn, Californian	see **Cascara**
		Bugbane	see **Black cohosh**
	48	Butternut	*Juglans cinerea*
		Californian buckthorn	see **Cascara**
	50	Cascara	*Rhamnus purshiana*
	49	Catnip	*Nepeta cataria*
		Catmint	see **Catnip**
		Chamomile	see **German chamomile**
	53	Chaste tree	*Vitex agnus-castus*
	45	Cleavers	*Galium aparine*
		Common chamomile	see **German chamomile**
	46	Common ivy	*Hedera helix*
		Cone flower	see **Echinacea**
	53	Corn silk	*Zea mays*
	52	Cramp bark	*Viburnum opulus*
		Cranesbill, American	see **American cranesbill**
		Culvers	see **Black root**
	42	Dill seed	*Anethum graveolens*
	45	Echinacea	*Echinacea purpurea*
	44	False unicorn root	*Chamaelirium luteum*
	45	Fennel	*Foeniculum vulgare*
	44	Feverfew	*Chrysanthemum parthenium*
	44	Fringe tree	*Chionanthus virginica*
	46	Gentian	*Gentiana lutea*

Corn silk is obtained from the silky pistils of the corn plant, Zea mays.

HERBAL MATERIA MEDICA

These herbs have been selected specifically for women's health problems, and to describe the characteristics of the herbs advised for various ailments. The "portrait" of each herb is necessarily abbreviated. If you become interested in herbal medicine, consider obtaining more specialized books (see p.186).

The herbs included here have wide applications and are frequently mentioned in the text of this book. A few herbs, of more limited use, are advised for specific ailments, but they are omitted from the list owing to lack of space. In such cases, refer to specialized publications.

Achillea millefolium
Yarrow

Parts used Plant.
Actions A general tonic, especially when combined with Hawthorn (*Crataegus oxycantha*). It warms the body and increases energy.
Indications Helpful for anaemia and general fatigue, such as after childbirth, illness, and radiotherapy (radiation treatment). Its warming effect soothes painful periods, and reduces excessive menstrual bleeding and menopausal hot flushes. Yarrow acts against other forms of bleeding, such as haemorrhoids or nosebleeds, and "breaks" a fever by promoting perspiration.
Dose To obtain the tonic

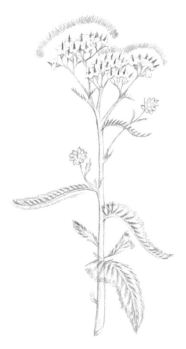

Yarrow is an all-purpose tonic that is helpful for a variety of period problems.

effect, use larger doses than standard. For example, take a 5mls teaspoon of tincture 3-4 times daily, in warm water if you feel cold, or in cold water if you have hot flushes (hot flashes).
Contraindications None.

Anemone pulsatilla
Pasque flower

See also p.67.
Parts used Leaves.
Actions Soothes the emotions, relaxes muscle spasms, clears mucus (phlegm), and brings out rashes and perspiration in fevers, so encouraging recovery.

Indications The tincture's soothing effects on the mucous membranes of the airways and digestive organs make it useful for coughs, asthma, and diarrhoea. It is also beneficial in problems related to persistent negative emotions, for example, those involving painful periods, delayed or scanty periods, vaginal discharge, prolapse, and irritability at the menopause.
Dose Take a lower dose than standard, at 2-3 drops of tincture, 3 times daily.
Contraindications None (but see Cautions).
Cautions All *Anemone* herbs are poisonous in large doses, especially when the fresh plant is used, when they produce inflammation and pain in the intestines. Do not exceed the recommended dosage.

Anethum graveolens
Dill seed

Parts used Seeds. The rest of the plant has similar properties, though milder, and can be used as a poultice for skin cysts.
Actions Promotes milk production, and is a gentle digestive tonic.
Indications As the "nursing mother's best friend," this herb increases milk flow; it is also a main ingredient in gripe-water, a digestive tonic gentle enough for babies.
Dose One 5mls teaspoon as a tea, 3 times daily.
Contraindications None.

Anthemis nobilis
Chamomile (Common or Roman chamomile)

See *Matricaria chamomilla*, p.49.

Artemisia vulgaris
Mugwort

Parts used Leaves. This common wayside weed can be found growing in towns, but avoid such plants, since their tissues may be contaminated with lead and other pollutants.
Actions Regulates periods, helps to circulate energy, and a tonic for the stomach.
Indications Three herbs with similar actions - Mugwort, Wormwood (*Artemisia absinthum*), and Tansy (*Artemisia tanacetum*) - are named after Artemis, the Greek goddess, because of their beneficial effects on women's problems. Mugwort is especially helpful for painful, obstructed or irregular periods. It also aids period problems at the menopause. The intensely bitter taste may be a disadvantage, but the bitter constituents are precisely those that assist the stomach.
Dose Pour the infusion into a bath, or apply a poultice of the leaves to your pubic area at times of pain. Take internally at the standard dose for 10 days before the expected date of your period.
Contraindications Avoid during pregnancy.

Cautions Do not exceed the standard dose. Large amounts over a long time can cause hallucinations.

Calendula officinalis
Marigold

Parts used Petals.
Actions Cools and soothes the skin; has various antiseptic properties.
Indications Used externally, as commercially available cream or ointment, for skin complaints. It cools and soothes inflammations of the skin, including spots, boils, sores, ulcers, eczemas, and warts. As an antiseptic, the ointment or infusion may be applied safely to cuts, and to sterilize the skin. Repeated application benefits varicose veins. A lotion from the petals soothes sore eyes and vaginal itching or soreness. Taken internally for painful periods accompanied by excessive bleeding, it encourages the heat to diffuse (see p.106).
Dose Standard dose.
Contraindications None.
Cautions Never use a tincture for eye problems, since the alcohol content causes severe stinging.

Capsella bursa-pastoris
Shepherd's purse

Parts used Plant.
Actions Stems bleeding, including menstrual bleeding; diuretic.
Indications One of the best styptics known to herbalists,

it helps to stop bleeding - without stagnation - in any body part: nose, lungs, bowels, haemorrhoids, and womb. In heavy periods it can reduce the flow without causing cramps, and is also beneficial in cystitis.
Dose Standard dose. Take for 10 days preceding each period.
Contraindications None.

Caulophyllum thalactroides
Blue cohosh

Parts used Plant.
Actions Tonic for the womb and helps to bring on periods; also a relaxant, antispasmodic, and diuretic.
Indications A general muscle relaxant, Blue cohosh is

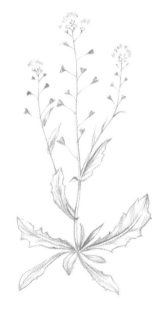

Shepherd's purse provides a remedy which is specific for heavy and/or painful periods.

marvellous for menstrual cramps, taken either when the cramps occur, or regularly for several months during the whole cycle, when it has a regulating effect. It is also helpful for delayed periods, particularly when accompanied by irritability and tension; for pelvic inflammatory disease (PID), to reduce inflammation and promote a sense of calm; and for contraction pains during childbirth.
Dose Standard dose.
Contraindications Avoid during pregnancy, except as a relaxant during birth.

Chamaelirium luteum (also known as *Helonias dioica*)
False unicorn root

Parts used Plant.
Actions Strengthens the uterus and lower part of the body; diuretic; relaxes and calms the mind.
Indications All "weak" pattern problems, especially anaemia, prolapse, heavy menstrual bleeding, infertility, watery vaginal discharge, and recurrent cystitis. As a stomach tonic, it relieves the "weak stomach" pattern of morning sickness in pregnancy.
Dose Standard dose.
Contraindications None.

Chionanthus virginica
Fringe tree

Parts used Bark of roots.
Actions Assists the liver; diuretic and tonic.

Indications An important remedy for a sluggish digestion, especially involving fatty foods, Fringe tree can refresh a poor appetite and reduce irritability, especially if you have a yellow-coated tongue. It aids recovery after severe diarrhoea, and gradually softens and dissolves gall stones.
Dose Standard dose.
Contraindications Since Fringe tree promotes the flow of bile, it has a laxative effect, and so should not be used during an attack of diarrhoea. Avoid during pregnancy.

Chrysanthemum parthenium (also known as *Pyrethrum parthenium*)
Feverfew

Parts used Leaves.
Actions Soothes headaches; encourages energy flow and lifts the spirits; strengthens and tonifies the uterus.
Indications Taken on a regular basis, Feverfew has the legendary ability to relieve or even prevent migraines (see p.176). It is useful for delayed or obstructed periods, especially when accompanied by cold hands and feet (a sign of energy stagnation) and after procedures such as D&C, or IUCD (contraceptive coil) insertion or removal.
Dose Standard dose.
Contraindications None (but see Cautions).

Cautions Large doses are purging, so do not exceed the recommended dose.

Cimicifuga racemosa (also known as *Actea racemosa*)
Black cohosh (Bugbane)

Parts used Plant.
Actions A tonic for the nerves and uterus, and a diuretic.
Indications Black cohosh has many applications, which stem from its tonifying action on the nervous system, and especially on the pelvic region. It helps nerve pains such as toothache and sciatica, and benefits "weak"-type pelvic problems such as prolapse, watery vaginal discharge, scanty or irregular periods, and urine retention, in particular when accompanied by a "bearing-down" or "dropping" sensation.
Dose Standard dose, but its action is slow and accumulates over several weeks, so be prepared to lower the dose after this time.
Contraindications Avoid during pregnancy.

Cypripedium pubescens
Lady's slipper (American valerian)

Parts used Plant.
Actions Relaxant and nerve tonic.
Indications This herb is similar to Valerian, although less of a relaxant and more of a tonic to the nerves. It is

specific for anxiety and apprehension at the menopause. It also helps stress-related headaches, irritation, and insomnia.
Dose Standard dose.
Contraindications None.

Dioscorea villosa
Wild yam

Parts used Roots.
Actions Relieves muscular spasms and acts as a digestive tonic.
Indications Helpful for abdominal cramps, either digestive or menstrual, and gallstones. Its specific uses are for morning sickness in pregnancy and for uterine spasms after childbirth. It alleviates anaemia when combined with other herbs.
Dose Standad dose.
Contraindications None.

Echinacea purpurea
Echinacea (Rudbeckia, Cone flower)

Parts used Roots.
Actions Transforms and expels mucus (phlegm) and purifies the blood; antiseptic and antibiotic.
Indications This powerful herb constrains conditions involving mucus or pus, such as spots and boils, erysipelas, and septicaemia (blood poisoning). In addition, it combines well with other herbs against eruptive or rash-forming diseases such as measles and chickenpox, and ovarian problems such as cysts and inflammation. It

boosts the body's natural resistance to infection and acts against most types of vaginal discharge.
Dose Standard dose.
Contraindications None.
Cautions Recent tests on animals by the US Food and Drug Administration have shown that massive doses can be harmful.

Equisetum arvensis
Horsetails (Bottlebrush)

Parts used Plant.
Actions Diuretic, drying and cooling; reduces blood pressure (antihypertensive).
Indications Relieves symptoms of kidney and bladder disorders, such as swollen ankles and urine retention, as well as nephritis, cystitis, and inflammation and ulcers in the urinary passages. Secondary uses rely on its haemostatic properties to reduce bleeding, as in nosebleeds or heavy menstrual bleeding.
Dose Standard dose.
Contraindications If there is high blood pressure, start with small doses, one-quarter to one-half of the standard dose.

Foeniculum vulgare
Fennel

Parts used Seeds.
Actions Warms the digestion and reduces griping pains and flatulence; promotes milk flow in nursing mothers; reduces mucus (phlegm); mildly diuretic.

Indications This gentle tonic can help recovery from illness or childbirth, taken as a tea or sprinkled on food. Its warming effects spread through the abdomen, helping to bring on periods and reduce menstrual cramps, especially in women who tend to feel chilly. The warmth also passes into the milk supply and makes the milk easier for the baby to digest.
Dose Use one heaped 5mls teaspoon of seeds for the infusion (tea). Make sure the water is boiling when poured on the seeds, and keep the cup covered for at least ten minutes while the seeds infuse.
Contraindications None.

Galium aparine
Cleavers (Goosegrass)

Parts used Leaves, seedheads.
Actions Diuretic; soothes inflammation in the urinary system; reduces congestion in the skin and breasts.
Indications This strong herb's most common application is for cystitis and urethritis, to cleanse the urinary system of poisons. It alleviates skin problems such as acne and boils, and the fresh herb makes an effective poultice for sore nipples.
Dose Take one 5mls teaspoon of tincture, 3 times daily; or one heaped 5mls teaspoon of leaves, as an infusion.
Contraindications None.

Gentiana lutea
Gentian (Great yellow gentian)

Parts used Roots.
Actions Promotes bile flow, cools fevers, and brings on periods; one of the most important and wide-acting herbal tonics.
Indications This tonic for weakness and exhaustion is particularly effective after illness, when the appetite is poor. Its bile-increasing properties are helpful for all forms of indigestion - especially "liverish" types, when due to overeating or difficulty in digesting rich foods. Other indications are jaundice (again as a bile promoter), and in combined prescriptions for anaemia, prolapse, and irregular or absent periods. A disadvantage is the bitter taste, which seems to inten-sify with repeated doses.
Dose Standard dose. Gentian is contained in the aperitif, Angostura bitters.
Contraindications None.

Geranium maculatum
American cranesbill

Parts used Roots.
Actions Drying and tightening; helps to reduce mucus, dry out inflammation, and staunch bleeding.
Indications Diarrhoea and diarrhoeal problems such as dysentery. Its drying qualities assist the natural blood-clotting process to stem bleeding of all sorts, especially from

haemorrhoids and the uterus, and it also has an action against urinary incontinence.
Dose Standard dose.
Contraindications None.

Glycyrrhiza glabra
Licorice

Parts used Roots.
Actions A general tonic that loosens mucus (phlegm) and revitalizes the lungs and chest.
Indications In Western medicine, licorice is used chiefly for mucus in the throat and lungs, and is an ingredient in many cough syrups and throat gargles. In traditional Chinese medicine, it is regarded as the "king of all herbs," superior even to tonics such as Ginseng.

With other herbs, it enhances their qualities and provides energy for them to direct. For example, Coltsfoot (*Tussilago farfara*) directs licorice's energy to the lungs, and Golden seal (*Hydrastis canadensis*) sends it into the digestive system, to cure gastric complaints.
Dose Standard dose.
Contraindications None (but see Cautions).
Cautions Excessive consumption over a long period can lead to raised blood pressure. It may also cause adverse effects such as fat deposition, similar to those caused by over-administration of strong steroid drugs.

Hedera helix
Common ivy

Parts used Pick the fresh leaves only, which should be prepared as described below, for external use on the skin (see Dose). Never take any part of this herb internally, in any form.
Actions A powerful astringent with cleansing properties; reduces pain and inflammation.
Indications The fresh leaves calm the nerves when applied as a poultice to the skin - for example, to the head for migraine, or to the lower back for sciatica. The cleansing qualities act against boils and skin ulcers, while the juice penetrates to nourish the skin's deeper layers; this helps to tone up slack skin, stretch marks, and similar "loose" conditions.
Dose With a food blender or chopping board, crush or mash a handful of fresh, previously washed leaves thoroughly with a cupful of warm water. Wrap them in a clean muslin cloth, and apply this muslin poultice to the affected part. It is best to pick and use ivy leaves on the same day (since the plant is evergreen, fresh leaves are usually available). If this is inconvenient, soak the cleaned, mashed leaves in vinegar, or lemon juice, or 40 per cent alcohol, instead of water. They should then keep for several days in the refrig-erator. However, do not

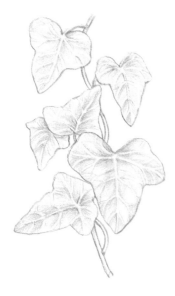

Ivy leaves (or ointment) help to smooth out stretch marks and keep the skin looking youthful.

use these preparations if the skin is broken, as they will cause pain and could be dangerous.
Contraindications None (but see Cautions).
Cautions Ivy should never be taken internally.

Humulus lupulus
Hops

Parts used Fruits, or cone-like strobiles.
Actions Relaxant and nerve tonic; soporific; brings on periods; diuretic.
Indications Hops' main use is as a relaxant and to induce sleep. Its effects on the nerves assist pains such as toothache, neuralgia, and stress headaches, and

anxiety at the menopause. This herb contains natural chemicals that are the same as the body's precursors of the female hormones, oestrogens, which possibly explains its use for painful periods.
Dose Take Hops as a standard infusion like other herbs, or by inhalation as a pillow or cushion stuffing.
Contraindications This herb can reduce sexual desire, in both men and women; this may be desirable or not, depending on the circumstances.
Cautions The flowers may cause skin irritation in some people.

Hydrastis canadensis
Golden seal

Parts used Roots.
Actions Works as a tonic and stimulant, and clears mucus (phlegm).
Indications This wide-ranging herb stimulates the digestion for sluggish and "weak" conditions (see, for example, p.98). Its special effects on the mucous membranes clear chronic mucus, especially when combined with other herbs.
Dose One-quarter to one-half of the standard dose (see Contraindications and Cautions).
Contraindications Avoid during pregnancy.
Cautions Initially it increases the amount of mucus expelled, so start with small doses.

Hypericum perfoliatum
St John's wort

Parts used Shoot tips, new leaves, and flowers.
Actions Drying and healing for wounds; relaxing and strengthening for the nerves and chest.
Indications The most frequent use is in ointments, creams, and other applications for painful injuries, since this herb acts rapidly on the nervous system. The oil-based extract assists healing of deep wounds and infected wounds where pus has formed. Taken internally, the tincture or dried herb helps to lift winter depression; traditionally it has been regarded as a "light-bearer." It also clears internal adhesions which may arise after injury or surgery. (It can be used homeopathically in the same way.) Other uses are for coughs and difficulty in urinating.
Dose Standard dose for internal use. Make the oil by soaking a handful of leaves in a cup of olive oil, and apply some on a pad to the skin. Pour two cups of infusion into a shallow bath, to help the perineum heal after childbirth.
Contraindications Avoid if you are very tired, when this herb can provoke rather than relieve depression. Since it is a "light-bearer" excessive consumption may lead to skin problems due to photosensitivity.

Juglans cinerea
Butternut

Parts used Plant.
Actions Laxative and tonic to the bowels; clears long-standing mucus (phlegm).
Indications Suitable for constipation, in both "weak" and "strong" energy patterns, although it takes up to 8 hours to work. It is also helpful in skin diseases.
Dose Butternut is a powerful purge in large doses, so take small amounts over a few months, to help restore regular bowel activity without a sudden reaction. Begin with 5 drops of tincture, 3 times daily, and increase this slowly.
Contraindications Avoid during pregnancy and when there are loose stools or diarrhoea.
Cautions Large doses are purging (see Dose, above).

Leonurus cardiaca
Motherwort

Parts used Plant.
Actions General tonic; brings out perspiration in fevers; calms and relaxes muscle spasms, especially in the uterine region.
Indications This herb is known internationally for its beneficial effects on the female reproductive system - its Chinese name, *Yi mu cao*, means "Help-Mother Plant." It is helpful for anaemia, various forms of weakness such as uterine prolapse, and painful or delayed periods. It

also calms the mind and reduces anxiety and panic, particularly when these are accompanied by heart palpitations.
Dose The standard dose is usually most effective as the tincture, or better still, the syrup.
Contraindications Avoid during pregnancy.

Leptandra virginica
Black root (Culvers)

Parts used Dried roots only; do not use the fresh plant.
Actions Activates the liver and bowels; promotes perspiration in fevers.
Indications The main use for this rather expensive herb is to cleanse the intestines and liver of thick, clogging mucus. Small doses gradually loosen the mucus and allow it to be expelled naturally; large doses are more violently purgative. The activating effects on the liver help it to metabolize poisons and increase secretion of bile, thereby aiding fat digestion and gall bladder problems. Combined with Quinine (*Cinchona officinalis*) and Fringe tree (*Chionanthus virginica*), Black root can assist recovery from postviral syndrome and other low-grade debilitating conditions.
Dose Standard dose, but in the case of postviral syndrome, take one 5mls teaspoon of the combined herbal tinctures, 3 times

daily. For gall bladder pain, as in cholecystitis, apply a Black root poultice over the affected area.
Contraindications None if the dried root is used. The fresh root contains possibly harmful substances.
Cautions In the first week of treatment, renewed bowel movements may cause flatulence and night restlessness. Large doses are purgative and should be avoided, especially in chronic diarrhoea.

Lobelia inflata
Lobelia

Parts used Plant.
Actions A wide-ranging relaxant that promotes perspiration in fevers; it is also an expectorant, emetic, and antihypertensive (lowers raised blood pressure).
Indications Lobelia's special effects on the chest make it useful in asthma, where it acts additionally as an expectorant. Among the many other indications are shock, trauma, croup, whooping cough, boils, high blood pressure, and tense, stress-related conditions, including migraine (when it may be applied externally). Its forceful action can overcome "full" or "strong" patterns of illness, for example in PMS (PMT, see p.90), painful periods, and excessive menstrual bleeding.
Dose Standard dose.
Contraindications Do not take

Lobelia if you are very tired or "over-relaxed," as in nervous prostration and paralysis.
Cautions This herb is restricted in some countries, and must be used under the supervision of a practitioner. In small quantities it may cause a temporary tight sensation in the throat, and perhaps slight nausea, but this soon passes. Large quantities are emetic.

Matricaria chamomilla
German chamomile

See also p.61.
Parts used Flowers.
Actions Generally a mild relaxant, but with a stimulant effect on the digestion; brings on periods and relieves period pain.
Indications This herb is commercially available as a tea in many areas, and its calming qualities make it a popular late-night drink. It moves a sluggish digestion, especially when there are cramping pains or colic. It also helps difficult periods, again when there are cramping pains, although it tends to increase bleeding (see Contraindications). The tea or ointment helps to reduce pain when applied to cracked or sore nipples.
Dose Standard dose; make the tea with hot but not boiling water, since the volatile oils are driven off by steam.
Contraindications Avoid if suffering from heavy periods.

Mitchella repens
Squaw vine

Parts used Plant.
Actions Well known for its effects on the female organs, as its name suggests, it strengthens and tonifies the uterus and pelvic region; it is also a diuretic.
Indications In preparation for childbirth, it gives tone and elasticity to the uterine muscles. It is helpful in all "weak" pattern problems (see, for example, p.98), such as period pains (when there is more of an ache than a pain), prolapse, excessive menstrual bleeding, and vaginal discharge. In addition it counteracts fluid retention, especially in the lower abdomen and legs.
Dose Standard dose.
Contraindications None.

Nepeta cataria
Catmint (Catnip)

Parts used Plant.
Actions Promotes perspiration in fevers; antispasmodic; calms the nerves; brings on periods; and is a gentle tonic for the uterus.
Indications One of the most effective herbs for delayed or difficult periods, including those of the "blockage" type (see p.123), especially when accompanied by agitation. Its antispasmodic properties ease the period itself. Its tonic effects on the uterus may help infertility.
Dose Standard dose, but the active ingredient is volatile,

so Catmint should be prepared as a tincture or hot-water infusion, never boiled. Take internally, or pour two cups of infusion into a shallow bath.
Contraindications None.

Nymphaea odorata
Water lily (Pond lily)

Parts used Roots.
Actions Strengthens the pelvic region; reduces sexual desire; eases inflammation in the genital area.
Indications An alternative to herbs such as Beth root and Squaw vine, this pelvic strengthener can be used for "weak" conditions such as prolapse, watery vaginal discharge, and weak-pattern menstrual disorders. Its cooling qualities tend to reduce sexual desire (in women and men). Apply the powdered root externally for discharging sores in the genital area. In some women it relieves the type of migraine that comes on before the period.
Dose Standard dose.
Contraindications Avoid if you wish to maintain or increase your sex drive.

Passiflora incarnata
Passion flower

Parts used Dried plant.
Actions Relaxes the nervous system; sedative and antispasmodic.
Indications One of the prime remedies for conditions involving mental over-

stimulation, such as insomnia, anxiety, and panic, especially at the menopause; and for nerve-type pains such as stress headaches and neuralgias. With other herbs, it can aid "weak heat" patterns of illness (see, for example, p.125).
Dose Standard dose. This herb is readily available in pill form from some pharmacies and many health stores.
Contraindications None (but see Cautions).
Cautions Do not exceed the recommended dose. Large amounts over a long period can dull mental abilities and cause headaches.

Populus tremuloides
White poplar

Parts used Inner bark.
Actions Strengthens and tonifies, especially the bowels.
Indications This remedy complements Gentian, which works mainly on the stomach and duodenum; White poplar acts farther along the digestive system, in the small and large intestines. It increases activity of the muscular digestive-system walls and enhances nutrient absorption. It therefore benefits poor digestion and loose stools, and its effects spread through the lower abdomen to work against conditions such as fluid retention, incontinence, prolapse, and vaginal discharge.

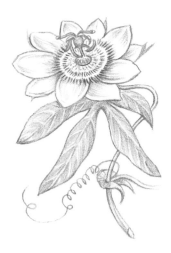

Passion flower acts to calm an over-stimulated imagination, especially during times of change such as the menopause.

Dose Standard dose; the infusion or tea can be used for a vaginal douche.
Contraindications None.

Potentilla tormentilla
Tormentil

Parts used Whole plant, including the roots.
Actions Astringent and antispasmodic.
Indications One of the safest and most powerful astringents, it helps problems involving diarrhoea and other discharges, such as heavy periods, vaginal discharge, cystitis with bleeding, and nosebleeds. Its cleansing properties are beneficial for skin eruptions and boils, and it is an effective gargle for throat conditions. As an

antispasmodic, it soothes cramps and so relieves painful periods.
Dose Standard dose.
Contraindications None (but see Cautions).
Cautions Large amounts may cause vomiting, so do not exceed the recommended dose. Do not prepare or use this herb with iron utensils, which alter its active ingredients.

Rhamnus purshiana
Cascara (Californian buckthorn)

Parts used Bark.
Actions As a tonic, it strengthens and moves the bowels, but large doses are purging (see Cautions).
Indications This remedy is still used in some hospitals as a laxative; however, small doses (5-20 drops of tincture daily over several weeks) strengthen the intestines and help "blockage" pattern conditions (see, for example, p.108), such as PMS (PMT) or painful periods.
Dose Standard dose or less.
Contraindications Avoid during pregnancy.
Cautions Large doses are a violent purgative, causing diarrhoea and vomiting. Do not exceed the standard dose.

Rubus idaeus
Raspberry

Parts used Leaves.
Actions Highly regarded as a uterine tonic, and energizing

for the other organs of the reproductive system and the lower abdomen.

Indications Raspberry leaf tea is an age-old remedy for pregnancy and birth, being especially beneficial during the last three months of pregnancy. It helps to improve the tone of the tightly-stretched uterine muscles, and relax away any premature cramps. During childbirth, it can reduce the pain of the muscular contractions without weakening them (see p.147).

Dose Standard dose, as a tea. This herb is also commercially available in pill form. The tea is recommended during childbirth.

Contraindications None.

Ruta graveolens
Rue

Parts used Leaves.
Actions Regulates menstruation; reduces milk flow in nursing mothers; works as an antispasmodic to soothe muscular cramps and tensions.
Indications Easy to grow or obtain fresh, Rue is recommended for "strong" and "hot" conditions (see, for example, p.113), including cramping pains before or during the period, when it should be taken for a few days as required. Taken over several months at lower doses, it brings regularity to an erratic or irregular menstrual cycle.

Dose Standard dose for period pains, and one-third standard dose for regulating the menstrual cycle. Do not boil the herb during preparation, since the active ingredients are very volatile and they will be driven off.
Contraindications Avoid during pregnancy, and do not take directly after a large meal.
Cautions Do not exceed the recommended dose, due to possible adverse effects on the hormonal system.

Salvia officinalis
Sage

Parts used Leaves.
Actions A famed herb with many and varied effects, yet gentle by nature. Sage is a tonic for the nerves and digestion; it assists wound healing; it is an antiseptic and astringent. In women's

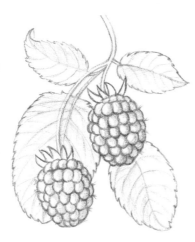

Raspberry leaf is a traditional remedy for easing the pain of childbirth.

ailments, it regulates menstrual flow and reduces milk production when this becomes a problem (for example, when weaning).
Indications Only a few indications of this wonderful herb, readily obtainable in most areas, can be mentioned here. It reduces period pains and regulates the menstrual flow, as well as helping to restore sexual desire when this is low through fatigue and exhaustion. Sprinkled on wounds, the dried herb forms a tough, flexible covering or "scab" that encourages healing. Sage tea is a digestive tonic for all "weak" conditions such as diarrhoea and excessive flatulence, and it also helps to strengthen the blood and overcome anaemia.
Dose Standard dose. Sage is best taken as a tea, but do not use boiling water or the volatile active ingredients will be driven off. Allow the herb to infuse for 20 minutes so that the bitter essences are drawn out.
Contraindications None.

Tilia europaea
Lime flowers

Parts used Flowers.
Actions Calms the nerves; antispasmodic for muscular cramps and tensions, and soothing for the digestive system.
Indications Lime flowers are an excellent remedy for easing tension and stress-related problems, such as

51

headaches. Migraine sufferers have been cured by drinking Lime tea regularly. It also soothes the nervous stomach and eases nausea and griping pains.
Dose Standard dose, best taken as a tea. Add hot rather than boiling water, or the volatile active ingredients will be driven off during infusion.
Contraindications None.

Trillium pendulum
Beth root (Birth root)

Parts used Root.
Actions Strengthens and vitalizes the uterus and pelvic region; works as a mild diuretic to increase urine output; and has related effects as an astringent.
Indications Beth root has been a traditional remedy among many peoples, including the North American Indians, for preventing miscarriage and easing childbirth (hence its common names). It brings energy to the pelvic region, especially to the uterus, when taken for about two months before the expected date of delivery. It also benefits weakness in the pelvic area, as in prolapse, stress incontinence, or watery vaginal discharge. The astringent effect reduces excessive menstrual bleeding.
Dose Standard dose.
Contraindications None, but inform your physician if you take it during pregnancy.

Urtica dioica
Nettle

Parts used Plant.
Actions General tonic; reduces excessive menstruation; mildly diuretic.
Indications Nettle is a general tonic and has a double action - it is particularly helpful for all types of anaemia, and it also reduces menstrual flow, being safe to take even during heavy periods.
Dose Standard dose, as a tea, or cooked in traditional fashion as nettle soup.
Contraindications None.

Valeriana officinalis
Valerian

Parts used Roots.
Actions Relaxant; tonic to the nerves and digestion; antispasmodic.
Indications This herb has a great reputation as a relaxant, and the tincture is widely available, particularly in continental Europe. Its chief benefit is that it relaxes without tiring; indeed, the relaxation it brings often produces a sense of vigour and clarity of thought. It is therefore helpful for migraine, nervous tension, insomnia, volatile emotions, and many types of stress-related conditions. It also relieves spasms and cramps, as in painful periods, indigestion, and severe flatulence.
Dose Standard dose.

Contraindications None (but see Cautions).
Cautions When taken in very large doses over a period of time, Valerian can dull the mind and cause headache and stupor. Do not exceed the recommended dose.

Viburnum opulus
Cramp bark, Guelder rose

Parts used Bark of roots.
Actions Relaxes spasms.
Indications As its name suggests, Cramp bark is good for cramps, spasms, and similar muscular problems. It works on any part of the body, but has a special and very rapid effect on menstrual cramps, often relieving severe pain in minutes.
Dose Standard dose.
Contraindications None.

Viscum album
Mistletoe

Parts used Leaves; the berries should be avoided since they are highly poisonous. Correct dosage is essential; large amounts are potentially harmful (see Cautions).
Actions Tonic to the lower part of the body; soothes nervous inflammation; antispasmodic; diuretic and antihypertensive (reduces raised blood pressure).
Indications Sacred since antiquity, this remedy has many uses. It gently calms and strengthens the nerves, banishing neuralgic and

stress-related problems. As a diuretic, it lowers raised blood pressure and strengthens the heartbeat. It is especially beneficial during pregnancy, when it can alleviate back pains and uterine spasms; and when breastfeeding, when it promotes milk production.
Dose As advised by a qualified practitioner.
Contraindications None (but see Cautions).
Cautions This herb must be taken under the supervision of a qualified practitioner. Large doses produce the opposite effect, according to homeopathic law - thus they raise blood pressure, and predispose to internal bleeding, miscarriage, and heart failure. The closely related species American Mistletoe is classified as unsafe by the US Food and Drug Administration.

Vitex agnus-castus
Chaste tree

Parts used Leaves.
Actions Regulates the menstrual cycle, sexual urge, and milk production.
Indications The common name derives from its use by nuns, to help control sexual desire. However it has many other applications, based on its ability to balance spiritual energy and sexual energy. If great sexual desire and preoccupation with physical sensations is a problem, it can help to open the mind to wider

possibilities; if reduced sexual desire is a problem, it can help to rebalance this aspect of femininity. Chaste tree also regulates painful, difficult, or irregular periods. Its balancing action may help overweight, when eating compensates for emotional insecurity. Other uses are for nervous insomnia, intestinal spasms, and controlling breast milk production.
Dose Standard dose.
Contraindications None.

Xanthoxylum americanum
Prickly ash

Parts used Bark of roots, berries.
Actions Tonic and stimulant, improving circulation to hands and feet; promotes perspiration in fevers.
Indications This remedy brings a sense of warmth to the stomach and intestines, due to the increased blood supply. It helps a poor or weak digestion, with swollen abdomen and flatulence. The widening effects on the arteries relieve cold hands and feet by restoring blood circulation. It is also a blood purifier and assists chronic rheumatism and cramps.
Dose Standard dose.
Contraindications None.

Zea mays
Corn silk

Parts used The flower's "silk" or "beard" (botanically the pistils, see p.41).

Actions Diuretic, antiseptic, soothing to the urinary tract.
Indications This mild tonic for the urinary system is beneficial for most urinary complaints, such as cystitis, urethritis, and pus or blood in the urine.
Dose Standard dose. Take every two hours for acute cystitis.
Contraindications None.

Zingiber officinale
Ginger (Green ginger)

Parts used Fresh rhizome (the familiar root-like underground stem).
Actions Warms the stomach and stimulates the appetite; reduces flatulence; an expectorant.
Indications Used for "cold" and "weak" conditions, especially weak digestion. It heats the stomach and counteracts "cold" and raw foods (see p.32). Ginger also benefits menstrual pain and obstruction of the cold pattern, when applied externally as a fresh poultice, or taken internally with molasses.
Dose Standard dose.
Contraindications Avoid in inflammatory conditions, since it can worsen these.
Cautions If taken in large doses (10 times standard or more) over long periods, Ginger can cause inflammation and weakness.

HOMEOPATHY

Homeopathy uses the energy and "vibrations" of remedies, rather than their material essences. It is based on the general law that a substance which is poisonous in large doses can cure in very small doses. This characteristic is embodied in the time-honoured phrase: "Like cures like." In other words, if the symptoms produced by large, harmful quantities of the substance are the same as those produced in the illness itself, then the illness can be cured by homeopathic (very small and diluted) quantities of the same substance.

Availability In many areas, homeopathic remedies and their close relatives, the tissue salts, are widely available from health stores, pharmacies, and suppliers of natural medicines. They are usually fully prepared and ready for home use. If you have trouble locating a supply, ask a local homeopathic physician or at a health store (see also p.187).

Preparation and potency

The mother tincture (for herbs) or the mother solution (for animal or mineral substances) is normally prepared in alcohol. This is then diluted successively in water by a factor of 10 each time. For example, 10mls of mother tincture is added to 90mls of water. One dilution by this factor of 10 is called a 1X potency. The 1X potency further diluted by a factor of 10 is the 2X potency, then 3X, and so on. Commonly used potencies are 6X and 12X.

At each dilution, or "potentiation," the liquid is "sucussed." This means the flask containing the liquid is subjected to very strong agitation, by banging or shaking it hard, to spread the remedy's energy

and vibrations through the preparation. Scales of potencies vary. In Britain, the most commonly used scale of potencies is the X scale described above, where dilutions are by a factor of 10 each time. In some parts of Europe the C scale is used, where the dilution factor is 100. Some practitioners use the M scale, at a dilution factor of 1,000 each time.

Throughout this book we advise the use of 6X potencies, unless stated otherwise. These are generally considered to be effective, yet safe; if you take the wrong remedy for some reason,' nothing happens. Higher potencies are stronger, deeper-acting, and longer-lasting, and they can produce unwanted results when used by the inexperienced.

Presentation Remedies are usually sold in the form of tablets, pills, pillules, or capsules. These are made of a simple, harmless carrier substance, such as lactose, that has been treated (sucussed) with the liquid remedy, to absorb it. Another form is the sachet or envelope that contains powder or granules, again usually lactose-based. Liquid remedies are available in some areas, and should be measured using the dropper technique (see p.39).

Methods of prescribing

Specific remedies are advised for most of the ailments in Part III of the book. In other cases, the simplest way of prescribing is to select a remedy by matching your own symptoms to those described for remedies in the Homeopathic Materia Medica section (see pp.57-69).

For example, the remedy Pulsatilla (which is related to the herb Pasque flower, *Anemone pulsatilla*) would help a

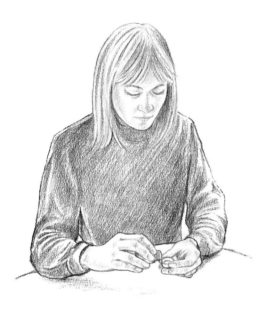

Homeopathic pills or pillules may be small and difficult to handle. After taking the cap off the container, turn it over and gently shake a few pills into it. Then tip the unwanted pills back into the container, so that the cap contains the correct number for your needs. This helps to avoid contaminating the pills by touching them with your fingers.

person suffering from a burning sensation in the throat, thick yellow nasal discharge, feverish cough, diarrhoea, and a tendency to tears. These are symptoms of an overdose of Pasque flower. Therefore, the closer the match between the remedy's symptom picture and your own, the better the results.

This principle of matching symptom pictures is excellent for acute attacks, and helpful for the inexperienced, but it is only an approximation. For better results in long-term cases, it is important to delve more deeply into the causes of disease. Homeopathic prescribing is

unlike most orthodox Western medicine in that it involves more than your physical symptoms. For optimum results it should take account of your whole being, including your tendencies, emotions, and life experiences.

Dynamics In long-standing disorders, the way a person reacts to an everyday event or situation is the key to successful homeopathic treatment, rather than the symptoms that result. It is thought that an inappropriate reaction to a problem in life leads to some form of bodily imbalance, which eventually manifests as symptoms. This concept is known as the "dynamics" of the remedy, and it is important for treating long-term, deeply-embedded problems.

For example, the remedy Lachesis includes several strong and unpleasant symptoms in its profile (see p.64). If these occur as an acute illness, it would be appropriate to take Lachesis.

However, the key for long-standing problems is not so much the symptoms, which are probably absent or vague in any case, but the situation causing them. Lachesis is especially useful for people whose personality and spiritual soul have become separated. Often they show cravings or compulsive talking, which reflect a much deeper need for fulfillment, and a need for the personality to be put back in touch with the soul.

For example, a woman who has been heavily involved in her career may be unable to find an activity that really answers her needs when she leaves her profession or retires. While the homeopathic remedy itself cannot change or cure her life, it can help to bring a new perspective that makes it possible for her to take the right decision.

Positive aspects In addition to the list of mainly negative symptoms, each remedy also has a "positive side." For many people, this is a novel notion - that every negative aspect of an illness has a compensating positive feature.

Consider a remedy with the positive aspect of generosity and a negative side of anger and resentment. Paradoxically, such feelings can coexist - you may be angry with one person, yet seconds later, show generosity to another. The explanation is that a warm-hearted person gives generously, but becomes bitter and angry if the gift is not appreciated. In this case, the correct homeopathic remedy can temper the generosity, so that gifts are given only to those who wish to receive them. So consider both the positive and the negative feelings when you select remedies - and you may gain insights into your own personality.

Constitutional remedies Homeopathy also includes the concept of "constitutional prescribing." It often happens that a person shows many characteristics of a remedy, but in a mild and long-term form. When he or she becomes ill, even with very different diseases, this symptom picture is accentuated. Therefore, if you prescribe from the symptoms, the same remedy is appropriate, again and again. This is termed the "constitutional remedy" for that person.

Constitutional type usually relates to a significant life problem rather than an individual illness. For example, you may (knowingly or otherwise) have difficulty expressing your feelings. Each time you fall ill, you could find that your symptom pattern matches that of a remedy such as Conium, which helps to bring feelings to the forefront of consciousness. This remedy would therefore help you in a wide variety of circumstances and illnesses, and you would thus have a "Conium constitution."

In this way, matching a remedy to a long-term problem is based more on underlying personality and "dynamics," rather than on the physical manifestations of symptoms alone - although the latter provide the initial guide.

Dosages and administration

For acute (sudden-onset) problems, take one dose of the remedy - one pill or powder sachet - every half hour for the first six doses, then hourly for the next six doses, then three times daily thereafter. You can continue for up to two weeks, but if the condition still persists after this time, consult a homeopathic practitioner.

For chronic (long-term) problems, take one dose three times daily, for up to three weeks; then miss a week before repeating the treatment.

When the remedy seems to lose effect, but it is still indicated by the symptom pattern, take 30C doses twice weekly, for up to 10 doses.

Do not take a remedy within 20 minutes of food or drink. Place it in your mouth and allow it to dissolve naturally under your tongue. For optimum results, do not wash it down with a drink or even plain water.

Caution While taking homeopathic medicines, avoid all coffee and peppermint, including peppermint toothpaste. These nullify many remedies.

HOMEOPATHY MATERIA MEDICA

This section gives a "symptom picture" for each commonly used remedy. The remedies are listed here in the alphabetical order of their international scientific names. There are many more remedies in the full homeopathic range, but limited space means we can only include those most useful for women's ailments.

To select a remedy, follow the prescribing guidelines on pp.54-56. Consider mental aspects first, then emotional, then physical. Bear in mind the Chinese principle: "In acute disease treat the symptoms, in long-term problems treat the cause."

Aconite
(Aconitum napellus)

Dynamics For situations when a strong force or event has affected your body or mind, causing it to put up a barrier. On the physical level, Aconite is appropriate for sudden chills, from a cold wind to an epidemic virus; mentally, it is indicated for sudden frightening events. Key features are anxiety or fear, chills, but without perspiration (compare Arnica).
Positive aspects Great alertness and awareness, heightened consciousness.
Symptom picture Mental outlook: fearful, restless, continually worrying.

Head: tight headache, with bursting pains; red, inflamed eyes that may worsen after

exposure to cold and wind; earache; sinusitis and nasal colds; sore throat.

Digestion-excretion: vomiting from fear, and morning sickness in pregnancy; scalding urination accompanied by shivery chills.

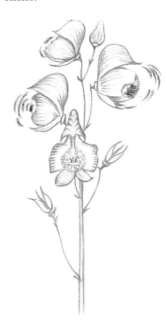

The monkshood flower provides the Aconite remedy. It resembles a monk's cowl held tightly around the head.

Chest: hoarse, dry, persistent croupy cough that comes on quickly.

Reproductive system: periods that are painful, delayed, or otherwise affected by fear; childbirth contractions that are painful or blocked due to fear.

Limbs: hot hands, but chilly or cold feet.

Sleep: nightmares, tossing and turning, restlessness.

You feel worse for: dry, cold winds; stuffy rooms in the evening or at night.

Actea racemosa
(Cimicifuga racemosa)

Dynamics Useful when your mental energy has become exhausted - for example, from too much study, business worries, or if you have worked hard and perhaps neglected your emotional needs. Helps to restore womanly feelings, and at the menopause, when pelvic energy declines.
Positive aspects Clarity of thought, putting your mind in control of your emotions
Symptom picture Mental outlook: claustrophobia and depression, at work or home; frightening visions or dreams.

Head: shooting or throbbing headaches, especially after worry or mental overwork; weak and sensitive eyes, with pains and dislike of artificial light.

Reproductive system: energy lack leads to scanty, heavy, or irregular periods, with shooting pains and "bearing-down" sensations; the greater the menstrual flow, the worse the pain.

Back and limbs: stiff, tense neck and back; stabbing pains in the lower back and legs from sciatica; generally fidgety and twitchy. Aching limbs, heavy and dull feelings in the legs.

You feel worse during menstruation, and when stressed or chilled.

You feel better for: warmth, which eases the pain.

Apis mel.
(Apis mellifera, Bee venom)

Dynamics When you do not deal with your emotions fully and openly as they arise. This may occur if you are preoccupied with one definite aim, and you ignore petty insults and difficulties, which then accumulate to a point when even a small problem hurts and "stings." These emotional features have corresponding physical signs of fluid retention and stinging sensations.

Positive aspects Energy, alertness, vigour.

Symptom picture Mental outlook: irritability from worry; grief, often with fear of death; muddled and apathetic thinking.

Head: swollen, stinging eyes, and possibly styes; stinging sensations in the throat on swallowing.

Digestion-excretion: fluid retention, involuntary passing of stools, burning sensations on urination.

Reproductive system: pain in ovaries, and either suppressed menstruation or very heavy periods with bright red blood.

Limbs: fluid in the knee.

Skin: burning sensations, and feelings of being pricked or stung.

Sleep: sleeplessness from worry; restless, shallow sleep; anxious dreams.

You feel worse for: heat, excessive touching.

You feel better for: fresh air and cool surroundings.

Contraindications Do not take during pregnancy. If cystitis occurs or worsens after taking Apis mel., stop the remedy (replace it with herbal ones) until the condition clears.

Arnica

Dynamics This is the "shock" remedy, that helps the body and mind to cope with and endure sudden, violent events. These include bruises and physical injuries; acute illness; and sudden disasters on the mental level, such as financial loss or grief due to bereavement, that causes numbness and dislocation (compare Aconite).

Arnica assists healing if taken before and after surgery.

Positive aspects Perseverance, without seeming to mind injury, discomfort, or fatigue.

Symptom picture The overall picture is of mental shock, yet a refusal to recognize anything is wrong. There may also be signs and symptoms associated with the cause of the shock, such as physical injury.

You feel worse for: being touched, drinking wine.

You feel better for: lying down, with your head low.

Ars. alb.
(Arsenicum album)

Dynamics This remedy has wide-ranging actions, and suits both sudden or long-standing conditions. It aids physical problems stemming from exposure to cold and damp, cold foods (see p.32), and food poisoning. Emotionally, it is helpful for anxiety and dread, and "cold fear" typical of the "weak" energy pattern (see also p.28). On the negative side, anxiety may lead to excessive tidiness, overwork, and perfectionism.

Positive aspects Neat and careful, reliable, dependable, ordered and organized.

Symptom picture Mental outlook: anxiety, fear, restlessness.

Head: pale face that flushes on excitement; headaches from too much study; itchy scalp; burning eyes; watery nasal discharge that burns the upper lips; hot sensations in the throat.

Digestion-excretion: indigestion with burning acid welling up into the mouth; sore stomach that reacts against cold drinks; abdominal pains and diarrhoea. Cystitis with chills and anxiety.

Chest: tendency to catch colds when the weather changes; night coughs.

Reproductive system: early, heavy periods that leave you exhausted.

Skin: dry, rough, or scaly, and worse with cold.

Sleep: disturbed sleep, with hands over the head.

You feel worse for: cold, damp and stress.

You feel better for: rest, lying down under warm covers with your head elevated and cool; the company of others.

Belladonna

Parts used Plant. The herb's rising energy splits into two or three branches instead of going straight upward, which is characteristic of the frustration that can be helped by the remedy.

Dynamics A constitutional remedy for those who have great energy and enthusiasm, but problems in finding a satisfactory outlet for it. It

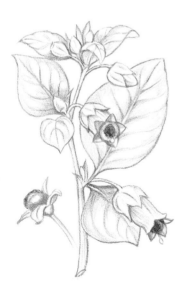

The Belladonna plant's rising energy splits into two or three branches.

counteracts "full heat" and "hot" patterns of illness (see p.27). It is also useful for the first stage of fevers (particularly from staying too long in very cold or very hot conditions), urinary infections, and uterine prolapse.

Positive aspects Full-blooded, energetic, enthusiastic, with a strong constitution.

Symptom picture The body is hot, red, and throbbing; symptoms may appear within 24 hours.

Mental outlook: irritability, desire to be alone.

Head: throbbing headache, worse on the right side and characteristically relieved by pressing on the site; red face; hot, light-sensitive eyes with swollen lids and dilated pupils; middle ear infections and sensitivity to noise; swollen, reddened nose but little discharge. Stiff neck and red, congested throat with tight or full feelings that make swallowing difficult.

Digestion-excretion: great thirst for cold drinks; stomach infections and sensations of fullness.

Chest: dry, painful cough that aggravates the headache; palpitations.

Reproductive system: early, heavy periods with bright blood; dry vagina.

Skin: dry and hot.

Sleep: difficulty sleeping; calling and grinding teeth.

You feel worse for: jolts and excessive touching, lying down, hot conditions.

Borax

Dynamics This secondary (rather than constitutional) remedy moves heat lodged in the system, that is obstructing your energy flow. It helps obstructed heat patterns of illness, especially when related to anxiety about losing your position in the workplace, family or community.

Symptom picture Mental outlook: vertigo and great anxiety, easily startled.

Head: headaches; hair tangles easily; facial pimples; red nose; sensitive hearing; sore lips.

Digestion-excretion: hiccups; poor digestion and loose stools; hot pains at the urinary orifice.

Chest: cough with gagging and retching.

Reproductive system: early, heavy and painful periods; white vaginal discharge that may feel like warm water.

Skin: scaly and dry.

Calc. carb
(Calcium carbonicum, Carbonate of lime)

Dynamics For situations when you feel lack of support, such as raising children as a single parent. On the physical level, it helps those with a constitution that is "fat, fair, chilly, flabby, and damp," who have a loose body structure, excess mucus (phlegm), and difficulty in digesting fats.

Symptom picture Mental outlook: "fragile," nervous, and frightened; easily depressed by life's knocks; forgetful and workshy; homesick when away.

Head: vertigo, dizziness from anaemia, and headache from overwork; puffy or chalky face; eyes hurt in bright light, and water in the wind. Noises in ears, ear discharges; dry nostrils.

Digestion-excretion: dislike of meats and fats. Appetite loss when tired; slow digestion and a tendency to loose flabbiness.

Chest: heart palpitations after eating; feelings of tightness and suffocation.

Reproductive system: periods that are early, long, and heavy, with sharp pains; milky vaginal discharge.

Back and limbs: chronic lower backache; cold, moist feet; arthritic lumps in fingers and toes.

Skin: soft, heals poorly.

Sleep: obsessive thoughts prevent sleep or intrude into dreams.

You feel worse for: cold and damp conditions.

Caution Do not take another dose of this remedy until the previous one has completed its work.

Cantharis
(Spanish fly)

Dynamics For times when passions run high (similar to, but more extreme than, Apis mel.). It is useful when you do not deal fully with your emotions as they arise, and they become too strong to overcome. On the negative side, this emotional build-up suppresses your individuality and creates burning sensations within. The remedy aids physical symptoms that are strong, progress rapidly, and involve burning sensations.

Positive aspects Strong positive emotions such as joy, enthusiasm, and abundant energy.

Symptom picture Mental outlook: strong emotions, high sexual urge.

Head: swollen, red eyes; sore throat and difficulty in swallowing liquids.

Digestion-excretion: vomiting in pregnancy. Burning stomach, worsened by coffee; sudden urges to defecate; painful, burning anus. Cystitis, with hot pains in the urethra and bladder, incessant desire to urinate.

Reproductive system: vaginal itching, sexual desire; problems in conceiving; early, heavy periods; vaginal discharge.

Skin: burns and blisters.

You feel worse for: drinking cold water or coffee.

You feel better for: rubbing the affected parts.

Carbo veg.
(Carbo vegetabilis)

Dynamics Strengthens weak energy flow and overcomes energy blocks (see p.25). For example, in acute conditions after an exhausting event, such as a fever, food poisoning, or childbirth, it speeds your return to health. In chronic conditions, it restores your enthusiasm and zest for life. Often indicated in anaemia.

Positive aspects A tendency to live in the world of the mind, thus a well-developed imagination.

Symptom picture Symptoms are explained by poor energy production and a slowdown or even stoppage of flow.

Mental outlook: irresolute; memory problems; little interest in surroundings.

Head: pallor from anaemia; dull expression and dribbling at the mouth; thin hair that falls out; dark spots ("floaters") before the eyes; nosebleeds, especially after exertion.

Digestion-excretion: slow, weak, and watery digestion, with swollen abdomen, loose stools, haemorrhoids, and pain after defecation. Poor appetite, choosy over food, "wet" vomiting, sleepiness after meals.

Chest: short, shallow breathing; weak cough; frequent sneezing and coughing.

Reproductive system: vaginal discharge; anxiety before periods; heavy, early periods but watery blood.

Limbs: weak joints, limbs "go to sleep" when still but revive on movement.

Skin: cold and moist, spontaneous perspiration.

Fever: normally cold and numb sensations inside, but

a tendency to perspiration after eating or resting, or at other unusual times.

Sleep: drowsy during the day but wakeful at night.

You feel worse for: cold air, fatty foods.

You feel better for: burping; gentle movements.

Caulophyllum
(Blue cohosh, Papoose root)

See also p.43.
Dynamics This remedy helps you to stay in touch with your femininity, and restores energy flow in the female reproductive system.

On the physical level, Caulophyllum eases muscular cramps and spasms, particularly in the womb during periods, pregnancy, and birth. On the negative side, you may have strong feelings and emotions that can overpower you and make you "stuck."
Positive aspects Great passion and sensuality, with a receptive personality.
Symptom picture Digestion-excretion: colicky stomach and abdominal pains.

Chest: spasmodic cough, tightness.

Reproductive system: painful periods; excessively painful and lengthy birth contractions; threatened miscarriage; vaginal discharge.

Limbs: joint pains in fingers and toes; muscular spasms in any part.

You feel better for: gentle movement.

Causticum

Dynamics For "dead nerves" and muscular weakness accompanied by burning sensations, often due to a profound emotional event (such as a bereavement or separation), that may prompt withdrawal from the real world. It aids weak contractions during birth, and is useful for a variety of problems in old age. .
Positive aspects Sympathy, a willingness to listen to the troubles of others and lend them support.
Symptom picture Mental outlook: sorrow, hopelessness, emptiness.

Head: poor or dim vision; noises in the ears; nasal discharge; warts on the nose; tendency to bite the inside of the mouth, greasy taste in the mouth.

Digestion-excretion: difficulty in passing stools. Stress incontinence.

Chest: hoarseness, pains.

Reproductive system: weak contractions in birth; menstrual flow lessens or ceases at night; low sexual desire.

Back and limbs: sciatica with numbness, worse on the left side; weak yet tense legs that tremble or "jump" and twitch at night.

Skin: sore skin folds; warts; old injuries re-open.

Sleep: drowsiness.
Caution Never combine Causticum with Phosphorus, since the two remedies have opposing effects.

Chamomilla

See also p.49.
Dynamics For problems due to high emotions - so much so that, if you are normally calm, do not use this remedy. If your strong emotions do not find an outlet, they bring on painful, cramping conditions and result in stagnant energy, especially when you are aware of the feelings. On the negative side, strong and deep feelings upset your energy flow and shorten your temper.
Positive aspects Generosity, warm-heartedness.
Symptom picture Mental outlook: impatient, irritable, intolerant, and quarrelsome.

Head: throbbing headaches or migraines; red face; earache; extreme sensitivity to smells; toothache, which is worse after warm drinks; bitter taste in the mouth.

Digestion-excretion: nausea, especially after drinking coffee; acid regurgitation; vomiting yellow fluid; abdominal pains and flatulence, worsened by anger. Loose stools that feel hot and painful. Cystitis.

Chest: irritable, dry cough, as if shouting.

Reproductive system: severe PMS (PMT) followed by heavy, painful periods with dark, clotted blood. Inflamed nipples.

Back and limbs: stiffness that improves with movement; weak ankles; cold hands and feet.

Sleep: anxiety and problems falling asleep, despite tiredness; desire to stick feet out of bed.

You feel worse for: warmth, anger, and cold, especially before your period.

You are helped by: warm, damp weather.

China
(Quinine, Cinchona officinalis, Peruvian bark)

Dynamics Emotionally, this remedy suits determined people who are basically generous, but who have become exhausted - perhaps by too much leading or entertaining others. It tones and strengthens after excessive fluid loss - from perspiration, menstruation, diarrhoea, and so on. It is indicated for long-standing conditions involving the liver; it also reduces the harmful effects of alcohol. On the negative side, you feel "liverish" and disagreeable.

Positive aspects Strong moral principles, great generosity.

Symptom picture Mental outlook: a tendency to be "prickly," seemingly trying to upset others.

Head: bursting headaches worsened by pressure such as brushing hair; bloated face that flushes readily; eyes with dark surrounds, yellowish whites, and dark spots ("floaters") disturbing vision; ringing in the ears; dry nasal mucus; toothache and gum pain.

Digestion-excretion: a tendency to digestive and intestinal blockages, causing indigestion, grabbing abdominal pains and vomiting; flatulence; yellow, frothy stools containing undigested food, made worse by fruit, milk, or beer.

Chest: dry, harsh cough that is provoked by anger or laughter.

Reproductive system: early, painful periods with dark clots; heavy feelings in the pelvis; bleeding between periods.

Back and limbs: shooting, knife-like back pains; dull aches in the flanks, limbs and joints.

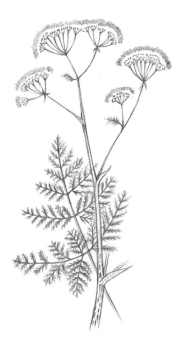

The hemlock plant is provider of the homeopathic remedy Conium.

Skin: very sensitive to touch; rashes and eczema.

Sleep: daytime drowsiness; racing mind and colicky pains at night.

Conium
(Conium maculatum, Hemlock)

Dynamics The remedy for numbness, either physical or emotional. Conium helps you to restore contact with your feelings, and face and overcome emotional problems when your emotional energy has withdrawn, as in mental numbness and "hurt feelings." It also is indicated for physical numbness or weak movements. Both are caused by repeated physical or emotional injury, or by long-term dissatisfaction that has been ignored. In addition, it is useful for enlarged or tender breasts, recovery after breast cancer, mucus problems, and swollen glands.

Positive aspects Resilience and endurance under stress.

Symptom picture Mental outlook: depression, a need to be alone; problems expressing feelings.

Head: bruised, dizzy sensations; easily disturbed by noise and bright lights.

Digestion-excretion: nausea, painful stomach spasms, mucus in vomit; symptoms improve after eating but worsen again two hours later. Weakness after defecation. Weak urine stream, possible incontinence.

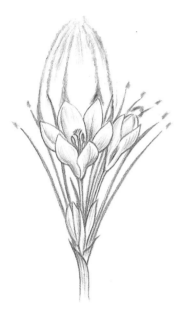

The "aura" or energy field of Crocus (Saffron) is strong, and shaped like a womb.

Chest: dry cough brings up sparse but thick mucus (phlegm); chest pains worsen when breathless or on bending forward.

Reproductive system: PMS (PMT) with enlarged, tender breasts and great anxiety; late, irregular, or scanty periods; other uterine problems.

Back and limbs: aches between shoulders and at base of neck, back bruises easily or even for no obvious reason; numb, chilled hands and feet.

You feel worse for: alcohol, lying down before or during your period.

You feel better for: moving about, eating less food.

Crocus sativa
(Saffron)

Dynamics For situations when you have an abundance of emotional energy - so much so that it can run out of control. Your feelings threaten the mind, with indecision and mood swings. The remedy controls and directs excessive emotional energy.

Positive aspects The overflow of emotional energy is a stimulus for others to get things done. With your aid, their self-worth is increased or restored.

Symptom picture Mental outlook: strong but alternating emotions; indecision; possibly hysteria.

Head: throbbing headaches, especially during the period or menopause; eye problems such as "seeing sparks," blurred vision, and a need to wipe eyes regularly. Nosebleeds with dark blood; lumps in the throat.

Digestion-excretion: fluttering sensations in the abdomen; constipation.

Chest: wheezy cough.

Reproductive system: PMS (PMT) with over-activity; heavy periods with clotted flow; "full" sensations in the genital area and breasts.

Limbs: cold, aching hands and feet.

You feel worse for: lying down, warmth, staying still.

You feel better for: being in the open air, rhythmic movements, creative activities such as music.

Gelsemium

Dynamics This remedy is suitable for both acute and long-term problems. It is indicated specifically for conditions or constitutions where the nerves are very sensitive and easily become overloaded, leading to weakness or paralysis (and also thick, grey mucus, or phlegm). Brings out the rash in diseases such as measles, and helps to regulate a healthy degree of perspiration in fevers. On the negative side, you feel easily weighed down and overcome by life's problems.

Positive aspects Great sensitivity and responsiveness; talent for performing arts.

Symptom picture Mental outlook: "stage fright," anxiety before examinations, and similar fearful reactions; this may develop into a numbing lethargy, with fear almost absent.

Head: dusky red complexion in fevers; heavy sensations, with pain at the back of the head; vertigo. Heavy eyelids, dim or blurred vision, bruised sensations at the back of the eye. Sneezing up thick grey mucus; a "dirty" taste in the mouth; difficulty in swallowing food, sensation of a lump in the throat, swollen tonsils.

Digestion-excretion: a dry mouth yet no thirst; diarrhoea. Profuse, clear urine.

Chest: heart seems almost to stop during exercise; cough, with thick mucus.

Reproductive system: late, painful periods; cramps in the womb and vagina; thick vaginal discharge.

Limbs: muscular weakness, trembling.

Skin: hot and dry.

Sleep: insomnia from exhaustion, obsessive thoughts, nervous irritation, and excitement.

You feel worse for: damp conditions, excitement.

You are helped by: passing urine.

Kreasotum

Dynamics For situations where your energy flow needs revitalizing, to banish weakness in the early stages of illness. It is useful for acute conditions characterized by accumulation and excess, and long-standing conditions where you are focused on the end result rather than the means. On the negative side, you accumulate violent emotions and their physical counterparts of discharges that burn and inflame the skin (compare Cantharis).

Positive aspects A strong will and deep determination.

Symptom picture Mental outlook: irritability, anger, wanting to be elsewhere; emotions relieved by music, perhaps tearfully.

Head: dull headache when menstruating; anguished expression; hot face, red

cheeks and lips; tendency to tooth decay, gum problems.

Digestion-excretion: nausea an hour or two after meals; foul-smelling diarrhoea, worse after curry, chilli, and other spicy foods. Bad-smelling urine, cystitis, sore bladder.

Chest: hoarse, painful cough with yellow mucus; chest pain and heavy sensations.

Reproductive system: great activity before periods, which are early and long, but reduced by walking. Vaginal itching, with yellow, burning discharge. Morning sickness during pregnancy. Bleeding after sex.

Back: dragging sensations, spreading down to the genitals and thighs.

Skin: itching, which worsens in the evening. Burning feelings in soles of feet, eczema on hands.

You feel worse for: cold air, winds, lying down.

You feel better for: warmth, gentle movements.

Lachesis

Dynamics Releases suppressed feelings in situations such as wounded pride, or in a conflict, as between parenthood and career. On one hand, strong but suppressed feelings may lead to compulsive patterns - too much gambling, drinking, sex, or work, and (on a more minor scale) compulsive talking. Physically, suppressed discharges may

lead to a dislike of being constricted. Particularly indicated for sudden bleeding problems, and postmenopausal conditions typified by the saying: "I've never been well since the menopause."

Positive aspects Mental alertness and agility, tireless and almost extreme devotion.

Symptom picture Mental outlook: weak-minded, forgetful; amorous, and intellectually gifted, but also jealous and mistrustful; talkative.

Head: headaches; eye strain; hard ear wax; nosebleeds and hay fever; toothaches; sore throat.

Digestion-excretion: compulsive eating; stomach tender to touch; haemorrhoids.

Chest: heart palpitations and irregular beats.

Reproductive system: scanty, lumpy, painful periods that ease as the flow increases; pain at the base of the spine during the period; painful ovaries. Swollen, aching breasts.

Back and limbs: back pain spreading to the legs.

Skin: bluish-purple hue, with boils, ulcers, and small blotches (purpura).

Sleep: sudden "starts" when falling asleep; symptoms worsen at night.

Lycopodium

Dynamics A wide-acting remedy for acute and chronic problems, that helps you to begin energy recovery when your physical, vital energy, and emotional levels have become weak (see p.14), leaving only your mind reasonably strong. Of benefit for premature ageing, in old age, and after any protracted and exhausting time, for example, coping with difficult children. For times when you may have lost hope and faith.

Positive aspects Kindness, friendliness, great endurance, and mental versatility.

Symptom picture Mental outlook: sensitivity, loss of self-confidence, dyslexia, sadness, and fear of being alone. Dislikes conflict, but takes out negative feelings on close friends.

Head: vertigo, dizziness on getting up; throbbing headache after coughing; grey-yellow complexion, with dark rings around eyes; difficulty seeing in the dark. Ear discharges, hearing problems. Keen sense of smell; dry throat, yet no great thirst.

Digestion-excretion: weak digestion, easily upset by foods such as cabbage, fresh bread, and onions; dislike of cold energy foods (see p.32). Swollen lower abdomen; diarrhoea or constipation from lack of muscular tone in bowels. Weak, copious urine, especially at night; stress incontinence.

Reproductive system: brooding before the period; sore, aching ovaries; heavy, late, extended periods; prone to "weak" uterine conditions (see, for example, p.97). Painful intercourse. Sore nipples.

Back and limbs: weak, sore lower back; weak legs; numb hands and feet.

Skin: lack of elasticity; brown or blue spots, ulcers, varicose veins.

Sleep: daytime drowsiness; twitching and waking at night.

You feel worse for: cold food, cold or stuffy surroundings, especially in the early evening.

You feel better for: movements, warm food.

Mag. phos.
(Magnesium phosphate)

Dynamics Soothes away muscular and digestive cramps, tensions, and spasms, which in natural medicine are often caused by cold conditions. This is mainly a remedy for problems on the physical and vital energy levels (see p.14).

Positive aspects Expansive, loving, and tender personality.

Symptom picture Mental outlook: laziness, apathy.

Head: vertigo; headache after mental strain; pain and stiffness in the ears, eyes, and throat.

Digestion-excretion: flatulence and colic, relieved by hot drinks; tendency to hiccups, especially after large meals.

Chest: pains, coughing.

Reproductive system: early periods; muscular cramps in the vagina, and in the uterus during menstruation.

Limbs: cramps, shooting pains, trembling.

Merc. sol.
(Mercurius solubilis)

Dynamics The "artist's remedy" that helps to restore depleted creative energy (see p.18), nowadays usually due to mental exhaustion from overwork. This leads to headaches, nervous and mucus (phlegm) problems, with putrid discharges, and in the long term, exhaustion and extreme tiredness.

Positive aspects Appreciation of beauty, adaptability, endurance.

Symptom picture A general feeling of dirtiness, with greasy skin, pasty complexion and bad-smelling discharges.

Mental outlook: loss of willpower, exhaustion; depression from thoughts of uncleanliness; even self-destructive tendencies.

Head: greasy hair, pasty complexion, spots on face and around mouth; thick, smelly discharges from infected eyes (conjunctivitis) and ears (otitis). Sneezing brings up thick, yellow-green mucus (phlegm); bad breath, unhealthy gums, throat ulcers and tonsillitis.

Digestion-excretion: flatulence, vomiting with much saliva. Blood and mucus in stools. Cystitis.

Reproductive system: anxiety before periods; heavy periods; thick vaginal discharge, often green or yellow; stinging and raw genital area.

Back and limbs: rheumatic pains, weak or brittle bones (see p.173).

Skin: profuse, greasy perspiration; spots and boils, sore cracks and skin folds; swollen glands.

You feel worse for: damp weather, overheated bed.

Caution Merc. sol. is for the strong constitution and Silica is for the weak one; they oppose each other and should not be taken together.

Nat. mur.
(Natrum muriaticum, Sodium chloride, Common salt)

Dynamics For those who have become emotionally exhausted, as a result of long-suffered feelings such as anger or grief, or from prolonged emotional output, such as nursing a sick person. The remedy restores balance and energy after long-term emotional involvement. On the physical level, it involves fluid disturbances such as runny nose, watery eyes, and fluid retention.

Positive aspects Reliability, independence, strongly defensive of others.

Symptom picture Mental outlook: a need to be alone; suppressed emotions, irritability; tendency to be a "wet blanket."

Head: headache before getting up; migraines with visual disturbances; eyestrain leading to headaches, and blurred vision; runny discharges from eyes, nose, and mouth.

Digestion-excretion: nausea, watery vomit; loose stools. Copious urination.

Chest: feelings of constriction, heart palpitations; watery cough that brings on headache.

Reproductive system: anxiety before periods, which are irregular and usually heavy, but with a watery, white discharge; prolapse with dragging sensations; dry vagina. Avoidance of sex. Withered breasts, nipple pains.

Back and limbs: weak, sore back; hot, sweaty palms; fluid retention and swelling in cold, numb legs.

Skin: greasy, with watery spots and eczema.

You feel worse for: salt, from being near the sea, or in foods and drinks.

You feel better for: fresh air, sweating.

Nit. ac.
(Nitricum acidum)

Dynamics For times when you obsessively pursue a goal single-mindedly, to the point where you ignore your emotional and physical limits. It is beneficial during or after middle age, when the physical body weakens and needs greater spiritual energy (see p.168).

Positive aspects Lively and vivacious personality, steadiness under pressure.

Symptom picture Mental outlook: irritable, vindictive, cold anger which may shock you afterward.

Head: rash from edge of lip; sensation of a band around the head; hair loss. Double vision and sharp eye pains; dulled hearing, yet great sensitivity to noise. Nosebleeds, greenish nasal discharge; bad breath, copious saliva, loose teeth.

Digestion-excretion: liking for fatty foods; burning pains in stomach. Constipation or diarrhoea, foul-smelling stools. Small amounts of smelly, cloudy urine.

Chest: harsh, dry cough; breathlessness on exertion.

Reproductive system: PMS (PMT) preceded by despair; early periods with heavy brown flow; sharp vaginal pains; vaginal itch after sex; withered breasts.

Back and limbs: sore back; sweaty hands and feet.

Skin: warts, ulcers.

Sleep: sudden "starts" when going to sleep; anxious, unrefreshing sleep with frightful dreams.

You feel worse for: extremes of hot or cold.

You feel better for: travel, by car or train.

Nux vomica

Dynamics Revitalizes if you have become physically and emotionally "stuck." Best taken with or after homeopathic Sulphur. Indicated for situations when pressure and tension build up, without relief from compensating physical exercise. The stress may lead to excessive use of alcohol and stimulants. On the negative side, you may feel thwarted and obstructed.

Positive aspects A vigorous, straightforward approach, with everything under control, and strong, decisive actions.

Symptom picture Mental outlook: confident of success, but irritable and finds fault in others.

Head: red, hot face; strong headaches, like "nails being hammered." Red eyes and dislike of bright lights; stuffed-up nose, hay fever; dislike of food odours. Sore throat.

Digestion-excretion: great hunger followed by indigestion; nauseated by rich foods when not well; nausea and vomiting, especially in pregnancy (see p.137). Constipation, with desire to pass stools but inability to expel them. Irritable bladder, cystitis.

Chest: sore, with a harsh, dry cough that brings on bursting headache.

Reproductive system: PMS (PMT) with hatred of partner; irregular, extended periods with cramping night pains, and dark flow; dislike of periods because they distract from work or other tasks. Sore nipples. Increased sexual urge.

Back and limbs: sore back; numb limbs which are weak in the morning; crackly knee joints; cold extremities.

Skin: hot, but easily chilled.

Sleep: wakes in the middle of the night, stays wide awake until dawn; sexual dreams.

You feel worse for: too much mental effort or moving about, rich or spicy foods, dry weather.

You feel better for: a brief nap, especially in the evening.

Phosphorus

Dynamics Overcomes "weak heat" patterns of illness characterized by red cheeks, restlessness, bright red blood, and dislike of hot, stuffy rooms. Causes of weak heat include lack of sleep, overwork, and excessive use of stimulants. These are related to nerve activity, resulting in great sensitivity - to lights, sounds, the feelings of others, and psychic activity. On the negative side you may be irritable and easily depressed.

Positive aspects Warmth, compassion, a truly caring nature; touching and skin contact is welcomed.

Symptom picture Mental outlook: depression, easily startled, fretful.

Head: dry scalp and dandruff; red cheeks. Great sensitivity to light, dim vision, dark spots

("floaters") disturb vision; poor hearing, especially for the human voice. Tendency to nosebleeds; burning throat.

Digestion-excretion: thirst for cold water; hot sensations in stomach; hunger soon after eating; forceful vomiting.

Chest: painful, dry cough, worse when with strangers, and the coughed-out breath has an unusual odour.

Reproductive system: tearful before periods; early, extended, but light periods with bright red flow; breakthrough bleeding; burning vaginal discharge.

Back and limbs: sore back, weak bones (see p.173), heavy hands and feet. Weak, numb limbs.

Skin: dry, bleeds easily.

Sleep: difficulty going to sleep, mind racing; dreams of fire; easily woken.

You feel worse for: being touched, exhaustion, hot conditions.

You feel better for: dim lights, cold food, cool air.

Pulsatilla
(Anemone pulsatilla)

Dynamics A "feminine" remedy for situations that women often find themselves in, due to an over-developed desire to please coupled with strong emotions. It balances the emotions with the will, so that the former do not take over. Two main features are bursting into tears easily (although the

67

sunny mood soon returns), and changeability - of moods, emotions, and symptoms.
Positive aspects Optimism, adaptability, a supportive approach.
Symptom picture Mental outlook: timid, tearful, irritable, changeable; likes support and values relationships.

Head: pains, especially at the front or right temple; burning tears, conjunctivitis with thick yellow discharge, styes. Nosebleeds or thick yellow nasal discharge, and sinusitis; swollen, cracked lower lip. Greasy taste in mouth; yellow or white tongue coating.

Digestion-excretion: morning sickness; dislikes fats, and warm foods and drinks; food loses its taste, no great thirst. Much flatulence; aching stomach and swollen abdomen. Loose stools with mucus and blood. Burning sensations after urinating; stress incontinence.

Chest: dry cough in the evening and night, which loosens in the morning; greenish mucus or sputum.

Reproductive system: gloomy before periods; extended, painful periods with scanty, dark, thick flow. Tendency to miscarriage or breech birth. Burning vaginal pains.

Limbs: shifting pains in limbs; hot, red feet.

Skin: urticaria or other rashes; skin spots before the period.

Sleep: slow and sluggish in the morning, drowsy in the afternoon, yet wide awake in the evening.

You feel worse for: warm air, jolted or bumpy movements, rich foods.

You feel better for: cool, fresh air; continual smooth movement, sitting up straight.

Sepia
(Cuttlefish ink)

Dynamics Traditionally used by women to restore energy and self-interest, so that you receive as much as you give. It benefits fatigue and exhaustion, particularly from supporting others. This leads to the negative side, when generosity in support depletes your own energy, making you unable to show affection yet unwilling to take a break because of guilt. Physical indications are all weaknesses, particularly in the pelvic region, and for sagging breasts.
Positive aspects Generosity, self-confidence, a supportive nature.
Symptom picture Mental outlook: suppressed affection; tearful when contemplating symptoms; guilt, apathy, introspection.

Head: dizziness from anaemia; dull, thin hair; pale complexion; dark spots ("floaters") in front of eyes.

Digestion-excretion: weak stomach, nausea before eating and bloated (but not replenished) feelings afterward; yearning for sour foods and fizzy drinks. Constipation, tendency to rectal prolapse and stress incontinence.

Chest: heart thumps and races on exertion.

Reproductive system: confusion before periods; "bearing-down" sensations as though the pelvic organs are falling out; dry vagina; heavy menopausal bleeding. Cracked nipples. Hot flushes.

Back and limbs: weak back; jerky limbs.

You feel worse for: damp and cold surroundings, overwork, too much sex.

You feel better for: sleep, rhythmic movements, warmth.

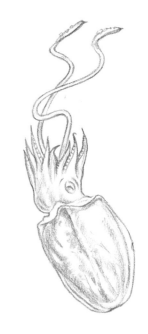

When upset, the cuttlefish Sepia throws out a cloud of ink to confuse others.

Silica

Dynamics Sometimes the balance between the will and the physical body is upset, making you feel vulnerable and afraid of failure. This remedy increases mental and emotional resolve and "fibre" and makes you feel adequately protected. Thus it is useful for problems where the will pushes the body and emotions to their limits, such as physical collapse, and for the early stages of colds, cracked skin and nails, and to bring boils to a head.

Positive aspects Strength, courage, resilience, the ability to pursue a project to conclusion.

Symptom picture Typical constitutional signs are a pale, thin, cool nature; vulnerable and afraid of failure.

Mental outlook: timid and tearful, with a tendency to go on until exhausted.

Head: headaches that worsen with hunger; sweaty head. Sharp eye pains, styes, and great sensitivity to light. Ears are similarly sensitive, with roaring noises. Nosebleeds and dried, crusty nasal discharges that bleed when picked. Gums and teeth sensitive to cold; gumboils. Sore throat and cough at first signs of cold or fever.

Digestion-excretion: poor appetite; great thirst but unable to take alcohol; indigestion and swollen abdomen. Stools difficult to expel; constipation before and during periods; tendency to stress incontinence.

Reproductive system: acrid vaginal discharge, itching; heavy periods with chilly sensations.

Back: weak, and sore in the lower parts and hips.

Skin: pale and waxy, with cracked nails and fingertips.

You feel worse for: cold conditions.

Sulphur

Dynamics A wide-acting remedy, with numerous applications. Its chief actions are against problems rooted in a tendency to live out desires in the mental world. This leads to anger, frustration, and "childish behaviour." On the negative side, you may be untidy and dislike washing, with the unsatisfied desires and anger bringing on physical itching and burning sensations - two characteristics of Sulphur.

Positive aspects The ability to turn situations to good advantage; jolly and jokey; intellectually creative.

Symptom picture Mental outlook: explosive anger, but then "forgive and forget;" depression, yet an active mind and vivid imagination. Sociable and sharing.

Head: hot, dry scalp, and hair loss; full, thumping headache. Burning, itching, red eyes; dark spots ("floaters") before eyes; whizzing noises and mucus in ears. Great sensitivity to odours; nosebleeds; persistent nasal mucus; dry, bright red lips; white coating over red tongue; sensation of a ball in the throat.

Digestion-excretion: poor appetite except for mid-morning snacks; foul-smelling burps; acid indigestion and aches over the liver area; tendency to hangovers. Hard, painful stools, haemorrhoids. Frequent, copious, sore urination.

Chest: continuous desire for fresh air; cough with much mucus.

Reproductive system: anxiety before period; late, short, difficult periods; vaginal itching and burning, with yellow discharge. Cracked nipples.

Back and limbs: stiff neck and upper back. Hot, sweaty hands; feet burn at night and feel better stuck out of bed.

Skin: dry, scaly, itchy and burning, as in eczema; sore, red, damp skin folds.

Fever: frequent high temperature, hot flushes.

Sleep: restless, talking, and twitching; wakeful in the early hours of the morning; preference for catnaps.

You feel worse for: remaining still, being too warm in bed. Symptoms worsen at mid-morning.

You feel better for: dry conditions.

EXERCISE, RELAXATION, AND MEDITATION

Since time immemorial, people have used physical and mental exercise to relax the body, settle the mind, ease pain, and cure illness. The Chinese text *Medicine of the Yellow Emperor*, written 2,500 years ago, suggested exercises for stiff joints, and meditation for worry and stress.

The physical-mental routines described here have been developed over hundreds of years, and they have many advantages. They require little, if anything, in the way of equipment and special facilities. They can be done at any time, and are completely drug-free. And they encourage you to focus your attention inward, to become more aware of your physical and mental condition.

EXERCISE CAUTIONS

● Above all, use common sense.
● It is dangerous to exercise while under the influence of alcohol, painkillers or other drugs, or while very tired or distressed.
● During your period, avoid exercises that involve being upside down, such as Neckstand, Plough, and Topsy-turvy. Menstrual fluid may trickle from your uterus "backward" along the fallopian tubes and beyond, which could cause a serious condition.
● If you feel sudden pain during an exercise, breathe in; then breathe out and slowly move to a resting posture.
● Sometimes you may have lesser twinges and aches, often described as "therapeutic discomfort." These come from stretching under-used joints, tendons, and muscles. Relax, then try again. But do not ignore repeated, strong, or painful sensations.

Which exercise routines?

First of all, choose a basic routine that suits you, taking into account your general fitness and the problem in question. Many exercise programmes can be used, not only for illness, but to improve physical and mental health.

Exercise routines and individual exercises with general application are included here. Exercises for specific problems are described with their relevant ailments, in Part III. All routines and exercises are listed in the Index.

If your energy levels are low (see p.25), consider the Easy stretch routine until you develop more energy with a stronger circulation. If you are very low in overall energy, begin with the Weak routine. This involves little energy expenditure, but it encourages correct breathing to take in adequate fresh air, and passive stretching to help the blood circulation.

For mucus and blockage patterns of illness, the Strong routine removes kinks from the body's energy pathways, encouraging a freer flow. The vigorous Dynamic routine also stirs up energy flow. If you use such strenuous routines, balance them with more static routines on other days. Variety in exercise is always a good idea.

If your energy levels are generally good, but local weakness is causing problems, the vigorous Dynamic routine should assist in redistributing your energy.

Always finish an exercise session with a relaxation routine (see opposite).

What should I feel? If an exercise is good for you, it should feel good, too. There may be a sensation of stretch, perhaps even some soreness - but this will have underlying relief and satisfaction. If an exercise seems too much effort, or gives a nasty sort of pain, it is probably not suitable for you.

Overcoming exercise inertia You may not want to start exercising. Perhaps it all seems too much effort - and will it really help? In fact, such "exercise inertia" often indicates an energy blockage pattern that by its very nature, makes you loath to become active. In this case, begin passively with the Easy stretch routine.

Relaxation routine

Have a blanket handy, in case you feel cold, and some cushions and books for support. Total time: 10-15 minutes.

First, sit up with your knees bent, buttocks and soles on the floor. Slowly lean back and let your spine uncurl onto the floor. Gently lay your head on the floor, arms by your sides.

Straighten one leg; after a few seconds, do the same with the other leg. This ensures that your lower back stays as flat as possible on the floor. If it pulls up, put a cushion under your knees.

Lift up your head in both hands. Look along the centre of your chest, and lower the top part of your head back onto the floor or the support of a few books.

Spread your arms at a comfortable distance from your body, palms upward.

Next, starting from the muscles of your forehead, try to sense and then relax the main tensions in your body - your jaws, the back of your neck, your shoulders, hips, and so on.

Take four long, deep breaths. Let your breathing subside. After a while, notice how thoughts come and go in your mind.

EXERCISE GUIDELINES

● Approach exercises with mental, emotional, and spiritual awareness. Respect the signals that your body and senses send to your mind.
● Do not be discouraged if you cannot follow the whole routine at the first attempt. Exercise, like other worthwhile skills, takes time and practice. Build up slowly.
● Try to observe the breathing directions. Worthwhile exercises incorporate free and rhythmic breathing.
● Do not force yourself to do exercises that feel painful or in any way unpleasant.
● Try to follow a main routine, in addition to your favourite single exercise. Slot chosen exercises into the routine as you wish.

Recognize that they change. Appreciate how transient and unimportant they are. Pay no particular attention to any one thought, yet do not resist.

Gradually, you should fall into an almost sleep-like state. Let it happen, but keep your thoughts moving along of their own free will. Eventually, refresh yourself with increasingly deeper breathing and some muscle stretching. Often a mere ten minutes' relaxing in this way can seem like an eternity.

As you come to, allow about 20 seconds for each of the following: roll over onto your side, put your palms on the floor and push yourself onto all fours, kneel on one knee, then put one foot forward and slowly stand with an exhalation. You should be refreshed and relaxed, and ready to get on with your day.

71

INDIVIDUAL EXERCISE ROUTINES

Weak routine

The exercises in this routine should require very little in the way of effort. Use your body's weight and balance to save energy. Breathe deeply, though, to take in fresh, energy-giving air. The stretching encourages your blood circulation to distribute the oxygen throughout your body.

Total time: 7-10 minutes.

Note: See p.70 for general information and cautions for exercises.

Knee hug

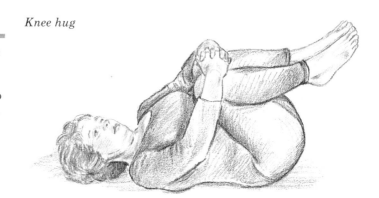

1 Long stretch

Lie on your back, fingers interlocked beyond your head and palms facing outward. Exhaling, stretch your hands away from your head and your feet and toes away from your trunk. With each new exhalation, stretch a little more, through the whole length of your body. Then relax for a while.

2 Knee hug

From 1, breathe in deeply. Exhaling, bring your knees to your chest and hug them with your hands. With feet off the floor, breathe naturally and let the weight of your hands sink onto your knees, to create an effortless, soothing stretch in your lower back. Remain for 60 seconds or longer.

3 Knee drop

From 2, lower your soles onto the floor and extend your arms sideways. Exhaling, lower your knees to one side, down to the floor. Relax thoroughly from your armpits to your knees. You may feel a sense of release at your hips and in your middle back. With each exhalation, let go a little more. Remain for 30-60 seconds. Raise your knees again, and repeat the knee drop to the other side.

Knee drop

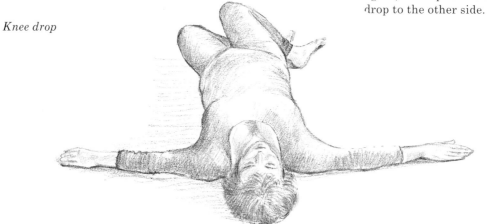

Weak routine

4 Cow and cat

Cat

From 3, roll onto all fours, arms and thighs perpen-dicular to the floor. Inhaling, slowly drop your belly down and look upward, like a day-dreaming cow. Exhaling, slowly arch your back up and look down, like a hissing cat. Remain for 5-10 seconds. Repeat each movement 5-20 times, moving gently with your breaths. Exercising your spine in this way helps you feel alert and tranquil.

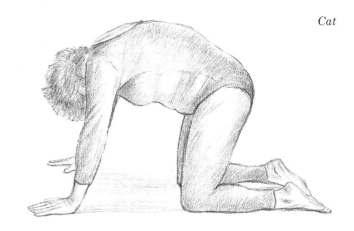

5 Sagging platform

From 4, straighten your legs to become a sloping platform, with bent toes on the floor. Exhaling, slowly lower your hips down onto the floor so that the platform sags. Remain for 3-5 seconds, letting go in your lower back and hips. Inhale as you raise your hips again. Repeat 5-10 times.

Cow

Sagging platform

INDIVIDUAL EXERCISE ROUTINES

Elbow hang

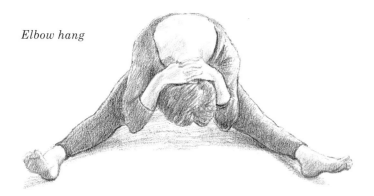

head to gaze at your toes, with head and feet making the two upturned ends of the "canoe." This releases tension in your neck and chest. Remain for 30-60 seconds. Finally, relax.

6 Leg stretch

From 5, stand in front of a table or stool, and place your heel on it. Relax, and create a strong stretch along the back of your raised leg. Extend the stretch up your spine by raising interlocked fingers above your head. Remain for 30-60 seconds. Repeat for the other leg.

7 Elbow hang

Sit on the floor with your legs apart. Interlock your fingers, palms on the back of your head. Exhaling, lean forward and let your elbows hang, weighing on your head, neck, and upper back. Remain for up to 60 seconds, breathing naturally. This releases tension in the lower spine, hips, and buttocks. As you exhale, slowly sit up and release your hands.

8 Canoe

Lie flat on your back, fingers interlocked behind your head. Exhaling, raise your

Leg stretch

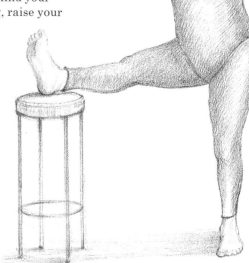

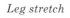

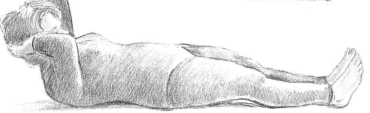

Canoe

Easy stretch routine

Easy stretch routine

This routine is helpful for gradually building up your energy, and for improving your suppleness and muscle control. If you cannot master the whole routine at once, develop it in parts, and gradually join the parts together.

Total time: 10-12 minutes.

Note: See p.70 for general information and cautions for exercises.

Leaning tower

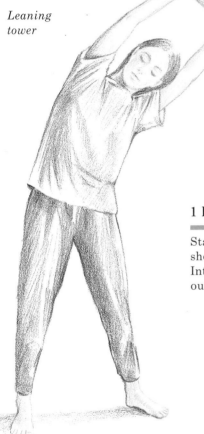

1 Leaning tower

Stand upright with your feet shoulder-width apart. Interlock your fingers, palms outward. Raise your arms high above your head to make a tower, and inhale deeply. As you exhale, lean loosely to one side, and take a few breaths. Then straighten, inhale deeply again, and lean to the other side. Repeat for both sides, about 20 times. As you relax, feel the stretch along your outer flanks and thighs.

2 Tent

Stand upright with your feet slightly apart. Lean forward, and breathing out, place your palms on the floor in front of you, with legs straight, to make an inverted V shape, like a ridge tent. Inhale deeply, then exhale as you sink your head and shoulders toward the floor. Feel your shoulder joints stretch and open. Aim your heels back and down to stretch your legs. Remain for 30-60 seconds.

Tent

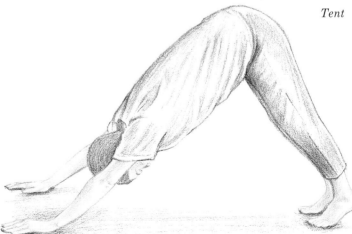

INDIVIDUAL EXERCISE ROUTINES

3 Cobra

Note: Avoid this exercise if you have back trouble.

From 2, exhale and lower your hips onto the floor, with arms kept straight. Point your toes backward, with soles up. Relax your legs, but tighten your buttocks and press your pelvic area onto the floor. Stretch your neck to look upward. Inhale deeply, filling your chest like a cobra's hood. Exhaling, push your chest farther forward, hollowing your back. Remain, breathing regularly, for 30-60 seconds.

4 Mermaid

From 3, exhale and kneel, sitting back on your heels. Slip your buttocks to the right onto the floor, so that you sit beside your feet. Extend your left arm across your front and put the left

Cobra

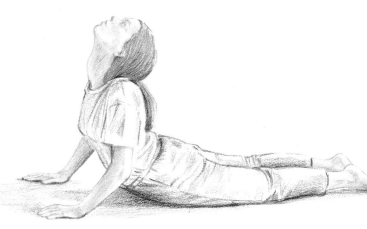

palm on the floor under your right thigh, fingers pointing inward. Exhale and move your right arm toward your back, resting the hand conveniently on the floor. Feel the stretch along your right side. Remain for 30 seconds, then inhale deeply. As you exhale, sit on your heels again. Repeat for the other side.

Back

5 Back stretch

(See also p.79.) From 4, sit on the floor with your legs straight. Hold your toes or feet; if you cannot reach, loop a cloth or belt over your soles and grasp its ends. Inhale deeply, opening your chest. As you exhale, pull your trunk toward your thighs, working up from the lowest ribs. Notice the

Mermaid

Easy stretch routine

Neck stand

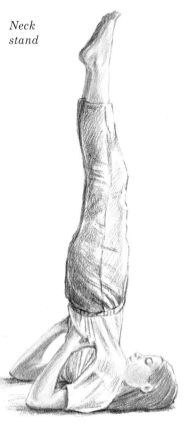

stretch along the backs of your legs, behind your knees, and in the base of your back. Remain for 1-3 minutes. Inhale deeply, and exhale as you slowly sit upright.

6 Neck stand

Note: Avoid this exercise during your period.

From 5, lie flat on your back. Exhaling, bend your knees up to your chest. At the next out-breath, hoist your back and put your palms under it. Exhaling again, push your trunk as perpendicular to the floor as you can. Straighten your legs to point upward. With practice, your body and head should make an L shape, standing on the angle of your neck, which you can hold for up to 5 minutes. Beginners may just relax into a more bent version for as long as you can, say 20-30 seconds.

Remember to relax and breathe freely. This deeply soothing exercise increases blood and energy circulation to your thyroid gland, in your neck.

7 Plough

Note: Avoid this exercise during your period.

From 6, try to lower your straightened legs over and behind your head. Rest them on a chair, and hold the chair legs as your knees sink onto the seat. Or you may be able to lower your legs so that your feet touch the floor behind your head, making an old-fashioned plough shape. This exercise stretches the spine and spinal cord within, lightens the pelvic region, refreshes your nervous system, and spreads energy to your reproductive organs. Finally, relax for a minute or two.

Plough

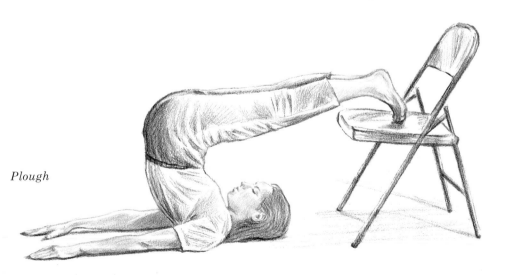

77

INDIVIDUAL EXERCISE ROUTINES

Strong routine

These exercises, although mostly static, invigorate the body and encourage energy circulation, as well as strengthening and stretching your muscles, joints, and tendons. They have a special effect on clearing energy blockages.

Total time: 12-15 minutes.

Note: See p.70 for general information and cautions for exercises.

Angle

Triangle

1 Triangle

Stand with your feet about one metre (three feet) apart. Point one foot sideways, the other forward and slightly in. Stretch your arms to either side. With knees straight, exhale, and bend and lower your trunk to the side. Go as far as you can, without leaning forward or backward, into a triangular posture. Point your upper arm to the sky and gaze at your thumb. Remain for 30-60 seconds. As you exhale, slowly stand upright again. Repeat the exercise on the other side.

Nose-dive

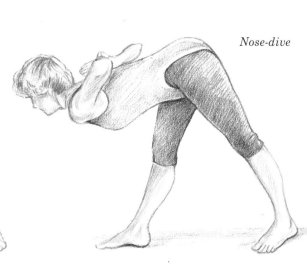

Strong routine

2 Angle

From 1, bend your trunk
sideways onto your bent leg,
and place the palm on the
floor beside that foot.
Stretch the other arm over
your head and against your
ear, at 30 degrees to the
floor. Remain for 30 seconds,
exhale, and straighten.
Repeat on the other side.

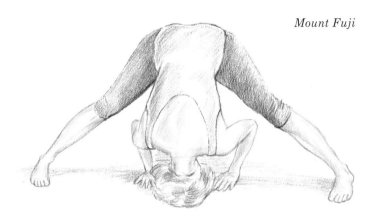

Mount Fuji

3 Nose-dive

Stand upright with your feet
one metre (three feet) apart.
Cross your arms behind your
back so that each hand holds
the opposite elbow. Turn one
foot sideways and the other
inward slightly. Exhaling,
twist your trunk to face in
the same direction as the
sideways-pointing foot.
Remain for a few seconds,
then exhale again as you
bend your trunk down
toward your leg, aiming your
nose-dive toward your knee.
Remain for 30-60 seconds,
stretching your buttocks and
knees. Exhale and repeat on
the other side.

4 Mount Fuji

From 3, stand with your feet
apart, toes pointing slightly
inward and hands on hips.
Exhaling, lean your trunk
parallel to the floor, looking
up. After a second, exhale
again while lowering hands
to the floor between your
feet. Exhaling once more,
press on your hands and curl
your head between your

arms, to form a volcano.
Remain for 30 seconds.
Exhale as you look forward,
and again as you raise your
trunk. This exercise posture
massages your abdominal
organs.

5 Back stretch

(See also p.76.) Sit on the
floor with your legs together
straight in front. Grasp your

Back stretch

toes with your fingers, or
hold a cloth around your
feet. Inhaling, pull on your
feet and look up. Exhaling,
pull your ribs toward your
thighs, starting from the
lowest ones; keep looking
upward. Remain for 1-2
minutes. This exercise
releases energy around your
sacrum and feeds it to your
reproductive organs.

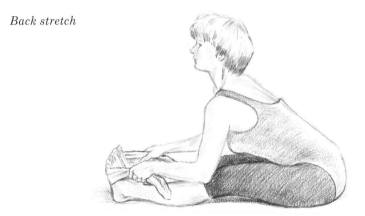

INDIVIDUAL EXERCISE ROUTINES

Dynamic routine

This powerful routine distributes energy evenly around the body. Although you do not use your legs, they should still feel energized afterward. Practise with the eventual aim of hardly pausing from beginning to end.

Total time: 15-20 minutes.

Note: See p.70 for general information and cautions for exercises.

1 Deep breathing

Sit cross-legged on the floor, back straight, and eyes closed. Place your palms on your thighs, with elbows bent and shoulders relaxed. Practise long, deep breaths through your nose. Begin each inhalation by letting your relaxed abdomen

expand like a balloon; then continue the expansion up into your chest. Exhale by letting your ribs retreat naturally, then deflate your abdomen. Continue like this for 1-2 minutes.

2 Belly rock

From 1, grasp each ankle with the hand on the other side. Inhaling, push your abdomen forward as far as you can. Exhaling, push your lower spine back as far as possible. Repeat with a

Middle rock

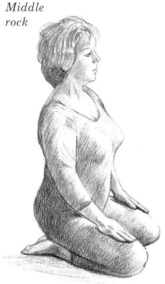

rhythmic rocking, faster as you warm up, for 1-2 minutes. Then go back to exercise 1 of this routine, before proceeding to 4, to allow any dizziness or muscular stretch to subside.

3 Middle rock

Kneel back on your heels, toes pointing backward, with your back straight and hands on thighs. Inhaling, push your lower chest forward; exhale as you push your middle spine as far back as you can. Again, build up speed as you rock rhythmically for up to 2 minutes. Repeat exercise 1 again before proceeding.

Wings

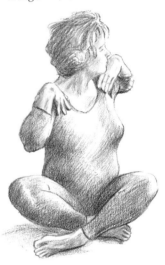

4 Wings

Sit cross-legged, as for 1. Grasp your shoulders, arms out sideways like wings, thumbs pointing back. Inhale as you rotate to the left, and exhale as you go to the right. Pivot at your hips, keeping your trunk as straight as you can, your arms flapping like a bird. Repeat rhythmically

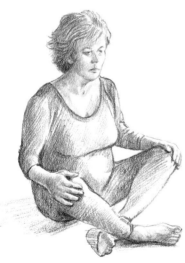

Deep breathing

Dynamic routine

for up to 2 minutes. This exercise loosens and stretches your lower spine, flanks, and hips.

5 Bear grip

From the cross-legged position of 1, hook your fingers together at the centre of your chest, one palm in and one out, "bear hug" style. Pull your arms apart hard while keeping the fingers clasped, and move your elbows up and

Bear grip

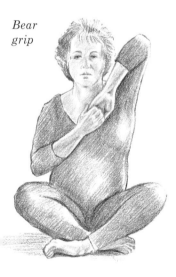

down so that your forearms rock in see-saw fashion, in time with long, deep breaths. Repeat for up to 2 minutes.

6 Chest rock

From 1, grasp the underside of each knee with the hand on that side. Inhaling, push your upper chest forward; exhaling, push your upper

chest back. Build up speed and continue for up to 2 minutes. Then lie flat on your back and relax for 1 minute.

7 Shrug

Sit cross-legged once more as for 1, hands palm-down on thighs. Inhaling, shrug your shoulders up as high as possible; as you exhale, throw them down vigorously. Continue for up to 2 minutes, building speed and breathing rhythmically, until your shoulder joints feel tired.

Neck roll

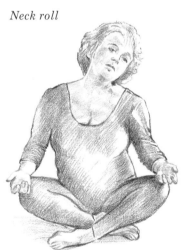

8 Neck roll

Sit back on your heels or cross-legged. Roll your neck very slowly in a circle, letting your head hang out and down throughout the process. Repeat 10 times, alternating directions.

9 Spike

Squatting down on your toes, raise your arms straight above your head, palms together to make a spike. As you raise your tongue to the roof of your mouth, inhale with a hiss through your mouth. Then momentarily jerk your upper abdominal wall back to your spine, before saying "Ha!" as you exhale. Repeat rhythmically for 3 minutes. Feel energy flowing up through your body. Finally, relax.

Spike

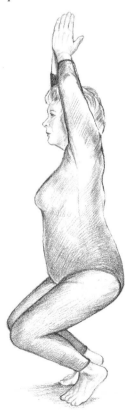

RELAXATION, MEDITATION AND THE ALEXANDER TECHNIQUE

The adverse effects of stress are well documented. Sometimes the source of the stress is clear, and you can do something about it. But more often, there is a vague and indefinable feeling that all is not well, and you can find no obvious cause for the problem. This is when natural therapies can be of assistance.

Stress is not a new phenomenon. The Chinese classic *Medicine of the Yellow Emperor*, written some 2,500 years ago, began with a discussion of the causes of ill-health. Near the top of the list was stress due to the "pace of modern life" (in addition to sex, drugs, and junk foods!).

Contemplation involves funnelling your attention onto an object, such as a flower. The tranquillity comes from creating space for yourself in a busy life.

In the past, people experienced severe stress, but it was mainly physical and dietary. They endured hardship due to exposure to the weather, poor housing, neglect of hygiene, and insufficient food.

In the West today, most people are relieved of the burden of exhausting physical work, and we are largely protected from extremes of weather. However, there has been a great increase in stress on the higher levels: emotional, mental, and spiritual. For example, from the emotional viewpoint, fewer people nowadays have the security and comfort which was provided by the extended family. We are surrounded by symbols of violence and sudden death, even including giant trucks roaring along the street. On the mental level, we are bombarded with ideas and sounds and images, often

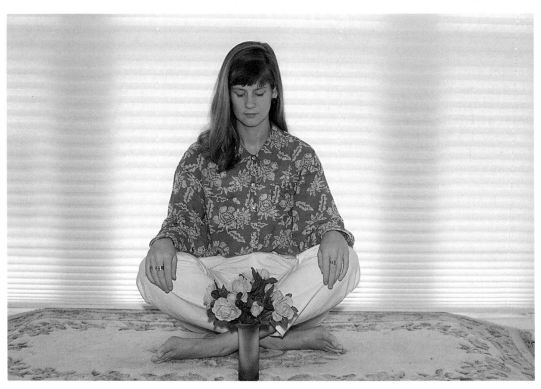

in lurid detail and of a most depressing nature. What can be done? An ancient Chinese proverb suggests: "A time of crisis is a time of opportunity." We need to become aware of the opportunities.

A book about natural medicines is not the place to discuss every self-help technique for coping with negative forces. We can, however, point out some methods to improve physical and mental health. These help you to build calmness and serenity into your life, and assist you in contacting your quiet centre of being (see p.16).

Relaxation

The simplest - and best - form of relaxation is to do something you enjoy. It can be physically active or undemanding, provided it is pleasing. Life's constraints are such that you may feel unable to follow your chosen activity or pastime. This is a missed opportunity. Make a conscious and considered effort to change your attitude, and relax by doing something you feel is pleasant, enjoyable, and fulfilling - for yourself, not necessarily for others.

One of the many effective relaxation and self-control methods is "autogenic training." These mental exercises aim to switch off the body's "fight-or-flight" stress system, and switch on the "rest-and-recreation" system. Autogenic training can be learned from books and videocassettes, and is also taught at many natural therapy centres (see p.187).

Meditation and contemplation

The purpose of meditation is to still the mind by focusing inward. Contemplation is similar, but attention is directed outward to a particular object, such as a flower or religious symbol. In the West, we have many opportunities for learning meditation and contemplation, from teachers and religious orders in most regions. If at all possible, seek guidance through the early stages.

The following simple routines, which can be done at home, give some idea of what is involved.

Loving kindness routine This routine helps to foster an attitude of love and acceptance. Each of the five parts should take about five minutes. Before you start, sit upright in a comfortable position, gently close your eyes, and relax.

MEDITATION GUIDELINES

If you wish to take up meditation, contemplation, or similar routines, bear in mind these points:
- Try to establish a regular time, so that the activity becomes part of your daily habits, like brushing your teeth. A good time is early in the morning, before the day's bustle has begun.
- Allow about 20 minutes. Less is too short for any real benefit; more may be too long initially.
- Avoid eating a large meal beforehand, which will make it difficult for you to concentrate. A warm drink and a piece of fruit or biscuit may help you to relax.
- Reserve a quiet place, and be on your own, without children, pets, or other distractions.
- The exercises should be enjoyable, not a chore. If you do not feel better afterwards, reconsider the situation.

COMMON PROBLEMS WHEN MEDITATING

● You may not be able to concentrate fully while meditating or contemplating, especially after the first week. You may be counting breaths, only to let your mind slowly wander - and suddenly you realize your 20-minute session is over! Do not be discouraged. This happens even to the experienced. Regard your mind as a child whom you are taking for a walk in a garden. You try to keep her on the path, but she tends to wander away. Do not become cross with her; instead, gently guide her back to the path.

● A feeling of black depression may begin to descend over you. Stop the routine. It may help to try another one, but it is preferable to seek advice.

● Constant interruptions from family, visitors, telephone calls, and so on are a common problem. The remedy is your determination. Once you persist for two or three weeks, you will be establishing a firm pattern.

● If a breathing exercise seems to fight against your normal way of breathing, stop at once and seek advice.

● Occasionally you may be overcome by a wonderful and exhilarating sense of well being. Do not be disappointed if you cannot recover this feeling for a long time. We should not expect such "treats" too often.

● Above all, do not give up. The time you spend is more important than what you appear to achieve while doing it.

First, develop love and acceptance toward yourself. The attitude of loving kindness should start at home. If you do not like yourself, there is little chance of liking others! Visualize yourself and say in your mind: "Let me be well, let me be happy, let me be full of joy." Repeat this for a few minutes.

Second, develop love and acceptance toward a friend. This is the next easiest step. Imagine a good friend of the same sex and about the same age as you. Say to yourself: "Let her be well, let her be happy, let her be full of joy."

Next, develop love and acceptance toward a neutral person. This can be an acquaintance you see occasionally, such as a store assistant or librarian, but about whom you have no strong feelings. Say again: "Let them be well, let them be happy, let them be full of joy."

Fourth, develop love and acceptance toward an enemy. This is a much more difficult step. Begin by choosing someone you dislike only mildly. Look for their good points. Let your bad feelings surface and try to dissolve them by positive thoughts: "Let them be well, let them be happy, let them be full of joy."

In conclusion, imagine all four of you sitting together. Try to accept and love each person (including yourself) equally, saying once again: "Let us be well, let us be happy, let us be full of joy."

Meditative breathing routine Each of the four stages lasts about five minutes. Try to make them quieter and more still, as you proceed.

First, sit upright quietly, shut your eyes, and relax. Count your breaths. Try to breathe naturally, not in any special way, and mentally count the number of breaths at the end of each exhalation. When you reach five, start again from one. Do this for a few minutes.

Second, continue to count your breaths, in fives again, but count at the start of each inhalation. This may be more awkward.

Next, stop counting and concentrate on the breath inside your body. Breathe naturally and be aware of the sensations; as other thoughts come into your mind, gently push them away.

Fourth, concentrate on each breath as and where it first enters your body. It might help to imagine this as being at the tip of your nose, or the front of your mouth. As the stillness increases, allow it to envelop you.

Alexander technique

This technique emphasizes the unity of body and mind. Through mental attention, you learn to change your reactions to everyday life, which otherwise intensify the stresses of living. The guiding principle of its founder, F M Alexander, is "conscious control." This depends first on stopping habitual reactions, and then on replacing them by more appropriate responses. The postural relationship between the head and neck is of utmost importance, in order to develop "good use" - good energy flow through the body. Alexander's discoveries have been supported by recent scientific research into nerve-muscle responses.

Many people attend for lessons in the Alexander technique when in pain, and use it successfully to relieve illness and suffering. But its best application is for those who wish to improve their postural alignment and acquire "good use of body." For this reason the technique is learned by students of music and drama, by devotees of yoga, and by athletes - all of whom depend on a high standard of mind-body coordination.

The role of over-exertion "Functional" medical problems (see p.12) respond well to Alexander training, since they often stem from inappropriate reactions to the stresses and strains of life. These feed immediately into the muscular system, putting the body out of alignment.

To compound the problem, our society emphasizes the expenditure of effort, rather than what is achieved. Often, we no longer notice whether the degree of force we use is appropriate to the situation. When we bring force to a task, we also force ourselves. The body is subjected to unnatural compression, which Alexander teachers call "Pulling Down." We do not sense this excessive force, or where our bodies are storing the tensions.

With the Alexander technique, your whole outlook can change: as your mind-body coordination improves, you become more responsive and calmer. People are often astonished to recognize the extent of their over-exertion, which reduces potential and may even cause harm. When you are released from this over-exertion, you feel light and free.

The Alexander technique has no religious overtones; it is strictly practical and can be applied to everyday problems. It can also be combined with other therapies. It should be learned from registered teachers who have undergone the appropriate training. Lessons are usually taken individually, although introductory sessions may be held for small groups (see p.186).

Part III

TREATING CONDITIONS AND AILMENTS

Home treatment by natural medicines is perfectly feasible for a wide range of illnesses and other problems. Yet for many people, using natural medicines represents a step into the unknown. They are more used to visiting the doctor, having a diagnosis made, obtaining a bottle of pills from the pharmacist, and taking these as directed.

However, if you make the effort, you will soon come to understand how natural medicines work, and how the powers of the different remedies and techniques can be recognized and harnessed. And, because you are taking on some of the responsibility for your condition, you are more likely to become involved, and to develop a greater understanding of your physical state, general constitution, and emotional temperament.

Using this approach, you soon become "tuned in" to detect the early signs that your body and mind send out, as ill health develops. You monitor your progress more closely, and you derive greater satisfaction in the relief and happiness of recovery, knowing that your own actions contributed to your return to good health.

CAUTIONS

Natural medicines can treat a wide range of conditions and ailments. However, many women (and men) have not had the chance to develop expertise in their use. In some cases, they have "handed over" their health care to the medical profession, and they have lost touch with their bodies and their mental, emotional, and spiritual awareness.

Times are changing, but slowly. Therefore, it is wise to seek the advice of a qualified physician:
■ to confirm a confusing, obscure, or unclear diagnosis,
■ to check complications are not setting in,
■ to assess any sudden or unexplained deterioration in your general condition, and
■ to deal with any life-threatening emergency as it arises.

Organization and use

This part of the book is divided into six main sections. Each section groups together ailments with features in common, as explained in the section introductions. Use of this material is explained on p.10, and a full listing of the ailments and conditions is found in the Contents (see pp.6-7). Or you can refer to the main Index (see p.188) for more detailed information.

It is also possible to select a treatment from the lists of remedies in the second part of the book. In addition, remember that most of the exercises can be used in combination with any therapy, natural or orthodox.

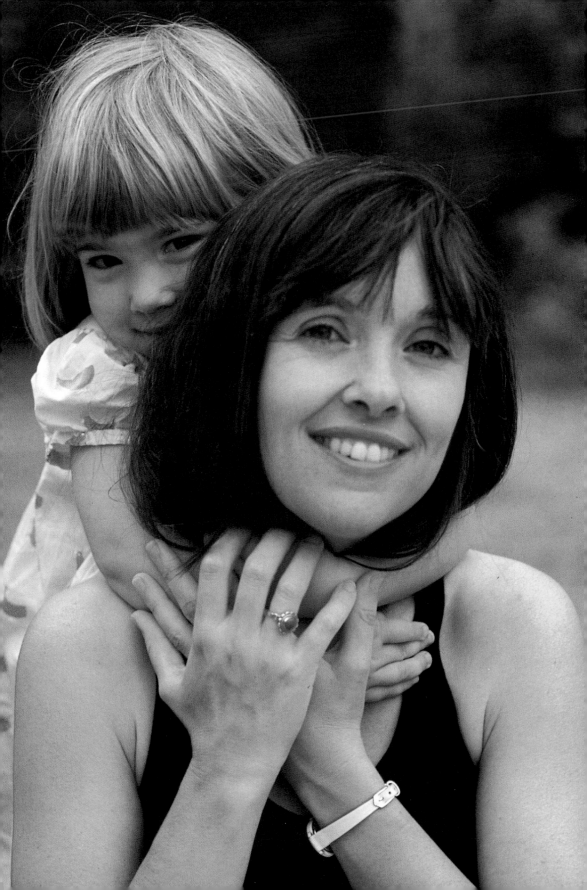

Conditions associated with Menstruation

For convenience, the menstrual cycle is usually divided into four phases: menstruation, before ovulation, ovulation, and before menstruation. It is normal for this monthly (usually 28-day) cycle to bring changes in your energy levels and emotions, as well as physical events such as the period (menstrual blood flow) itself.

This section of the book outlines the normal pattern of changes that takes place, and how and why things may go wrong. Familiarity with the normal pattern will open the way for greater understanding of your own responses during the cycle.

Energy changes at menstruation

The onset of menstruation marks both the end of one cycle and the beginning of the next. It is a time of great importance, when you may feel that your sense of identity and individuality is at its most intense. Your energy is farthest away from the physical level, and closest to the source of all life, so that enough "spirit" can be drawn down for conception (see p.127).

The beginning of the new marks the end of the old, with the outflow of unused matter that had accumulated during the previous cycle. With it goes any build-up of toxins (poisons) on the physical level, and also any emotional dregs that have collected over the month. In this way your body and mind are purified and cleansed, ready for the new input of spiritual energy.

At this time, too, you may feel yourself reaching "upward" to meet the renewed spiritual energy. You may feel distant from everyday life, perhaps less ordered in your regular activities, and prone to fainting. This so-called irrational behaviour would be better called "instinctual," however, for you may be hearing your quiet inner voice with greater clarity. It is a time to feel free, and to follow your natural feelings and intuitions.

Most women have a strong and instinctive dislike of making love at this time. Sex has the effect of "grounding" them and taking them away from contact with the spiritual source. Others have increased sexual feelings at this time.

Energy changes after menstruation

In the two weeks or so after menstruation, your body becomes ready to create a new life, to nurture it, and to provide the physical environment within which it can grow. Your renewed spiritual energy is drawn downward, day by day, through the emotional layers to the physical level. Thus, at ovulation time, your consciousness has become focused on the physical. In Chinese medicine, the womb "does its work" during these two weeks. The body's energy and blood are directed more and more to the womb, peaking at ovulation time.

If you are strong and vigorous, you may feel at your most comfortable during these two weeks. But if you are short of energy or anaemic, this can be the most difficult part of the cycle. The womb takes a great proportion of the body's energy, which may be in short supply, thereby aggravating any problems.

Energy changes at ovulation

Ovulation is the "opposite" part of the cycle to menstruation, and energy levels take up the opposing configuration.

Physical energy is strong, and spiritual energy has declined. Your consciousness may well be at its most materialistic and physical during this time, which is often reflected in a greater degree of sexual activity. You may also feel at your most feminine, with an abundance of the "female" Yin energy.

A common physical counterpart of these energy changes is a slight milky, perhaps sticky, discharge from the uterus and vagina. Some women have slight abdominal pain in the middle of the cycle, due either to obstruction of the normal flow of these fluids or to ovulation.

Energy changes before menstruation

Immediately after ovulation, the womb is at its fullest, ready to receive a new life. It is waiting and still. If conception takes place, then the new spirit will draw on the accumulated reserves. If there is no conception, then the waiting goes on. In Chinese medicine, it is said that the womb "rests" at this stage. If you are strong and vigorous, you may view the resting and waiting as an irritation and nuisance, especially if you live an active and creative life. You may dislike the sensation of your consciousness gradually withdrawing from the physical world, back up toward the spiritual level.

As the cycle started, so it ends - with menstruation. Inconvenient and painful it may be, but the spiritual energy that you instinctively contact at this time can benefit both you and those around you.

The four main phases of the menstrual cycle are accompanied by a change in the focus of energy. It moves from the basic physical level during ovulation, to the higher spiritual plane during menstruation.

Spiritual level

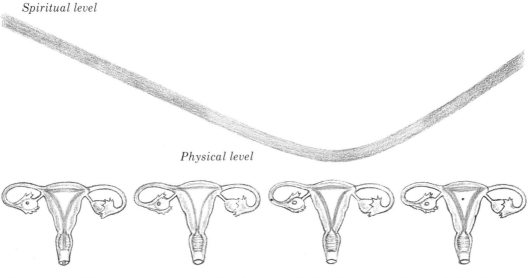

Physical level

Menstruation rids the body of toxins and emotional dregs

After menstruation, the womb prepares to nurture a new life

At ovulation, the lining of the womb is thickened and full

After ovulation, the womb "rests" until its lining fragments

PREMENSTRUAL SYNDROME (PMS or PMT)

Premenstrual syndrome (PMS), which includes the condition known as Premenstrual tension (PMT), is so widespread, and so many women fear the upheavals that occur in the days preceding their period, that the period itself is often called "the curse." This name tends to reinforce the negative aspects of the period, and obscures its more positive effects (see p.88).

Physical causes

Orthodox medicine attributes PMS to an imbalance in the hormones. In natural medicine, the hormonal imbalance is significant, but it is seen as part of a wider symptom picture involving an imbalance in liver function. (The liver is the main organ for dealing with toxins.)

During the days before a period, your liver prepares to expel any toxins (poisons) that have accumulated in the system, working vigorously in the same way as after a heavy meal or too much alcohol. This is why some symptoms associated with PMS resemble those of a hangover. It also explains why some women find that drinking alcohol can relieve PMS for a few hours, although the symptoms soon return - and they are often more severe. And it explains why coffee (even decaffeinated) gives short-term relief from PMS, but has long-term bad effects.

In some women, PMS is aggravated by an earlier illness such as hepatitis, that affected the liver.

Emotional aspects

A great difference between men and women is the cyclical nature of the woman's emotional energy, and this manifests itself most vividly in PMS. Although the tension and negative effects usually appear in the week or so before the period, they really result from an accumulation of all the tensions from the previous month (or in some cases years!). Feelings that can spark off PMS include irritation, anger, anxiety, and types of stresses that might also predispose to high blood pressure (although this is more common in men).

Life tensions The emotions, tensions, and other factors that give rise to PMS often come from an imbalance in the feminine side of the personality. This may happen if you work in a male-dominated factory, office, or similar situation, where you are subjected to the pressures of a "man's world."

Other factors that may contribute to PMS include an overcrowded timetable, so that you are always hurrying, or very strict, self-imposed standards of tidiness and order, which you may find difficult to maintain.

Mental and spiritual problems The origin of the emotional imbalance underlying PMS is often found on a higher plane - in particular, from a problem relating to femininity. As society changes, some women have difficulty in perceiving how to be feminine without appearing weak. The conventional wisdom - a product of a largely male-orientated world - deems that showing emotions indicates weakness, and that bursting into tears is unacceptable.

Consider this for what it is: the male method of self-defense, and of saving emotional energy. People feel embarrassed when someone shows their raw, vulnerable side and bursts into a rage or tears. They "stiffen" to protect themselves and resist the outpouring of emotions. This stiffening and resistance can contribute to PMS.

Symptoms

In mild cases the symptoms start a day or two before the period, while in severe cases they may start as much as two weeks before. They include:

■ tension, irritability, and depression,
■ bursting into tears, or suddenly flying into a rage over small things,
■ swollen, tender breasts,
■ a "full" feeling in the lower abdomen,
■ headache, and
■ insomnia.

Prevention

There are many ways to help prevent PMS. Some may seem obvious - but are you really acting upon them?

Avoid stimulants, especially coffee and tea, and not just before the period but all the time. Take Chamomile tea (*Anthemis nobilis*) as a regular drink. Stay clear of red meat, red wine, and fatty foods. Drink alcohol only once a week, if at all.

Try to live life at a sensible pace, without too much rushing around. Enjoyable exercise such as swimming or walking helps to get your energy moving, and so brings relief from PMS. If you often feel pushed beyond your limit, treatment will only be effective for a short while.

TREATMENT FOR PREMENSTRUAL SYNDROME

These treatments should have some effect if taken while you experience PMS, but the best time to treat it is before it occurs. Follow the advice for several months, and the positive effects will accumulate.

Herbs

Note: See p.38 for doses and cautions for herbs.

You should feel some benefit after your first course of herbal remedy. Continue for at least 3 cycles, and up to 12 cycles. If tension still persists, consult a practitioner of natural medicine.
● Take one Agnus castus 50mgs pill, 3 times daily for 3 months, even longer.
● Or take a combined prescription of the standard doses of these herbs, for 10-14 days before the period (ideally from the time of ovulation): Feverfew (*Chrysanthemum parthenium*), Motherwort (*Leonurus cardiaca*), Blue cohosh (*Caulophyllum thalactroides*), and either Valerian (*Valeriana officinalis*) or Lady's slipper (*Cypripedium pubescens*).

Feverfew moves the body's energy and improves the digestion; Motherwort is a general relaxant and hormonal regulator; Blue cohosh is specific for PMS; while Valerian and Lady's slipper are general herbal relaxants.
● If you have constipation, add Cascara (*Rhamnus purshiana*) to one of the above prescriptions. Start with a standard dose, and increase this by up to 5 times, as required.
● A mild herb you might try regularly as a tea is Catmint (*Nepeta cataria*).

Naturopathy

Note: See p.186 for specialist publications.
● Evening primrose oil and Vitamin B6.

Continued on next page

Continued from previous page

Homeopathy

Note: See p.54 for doses and cautions for homeopathic remedies.

Select one or more of the following remedies, as indicated, and take them during the 2 weeks before your period. Use 6X potency, 3 times daily.

● If you feel exhausted before your period, with a poor appetite, and perhaps

Temple guardian

an ache in one ovary, or cramping pains in the womb area - Belladonna.

● If you are very tired and easily startled, you feel chilly, and your breasts are swollen and tender - Calc. carb.

● If you are very irritable and restless - Chamomilla.

● If you suffer nausea - Nux vomica.

● If you have swollen and tender breasts, swollen glands, aching muscles, and your dreams are disturbing - Conium.

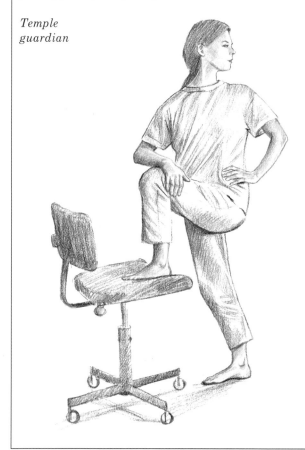

● Other helpful remedies include Causticum, Graphites, Kali carb., Kreasotum, Lycopodium, Nat. mur., Phosphorus, Sepia, and Sulphur (see pp.57-69).

Exercises

Note: See p.70 for details of exercise routines.

Carry out exercises daily, preferably the Strong or Dynamic routine. In addition, to break the strait-jacket mould:

● Temple guardian. Stand in front of a chair, and put your right foot on the seat. Place your right hand on your right hip. Exhaling, pull on your right thigh with your left hand, to twist your trunk around to the right. Look over your right shoulder as you do this, and hold the position for 30-60 seconds. Relax, face the front, and do the same on the other side. Feel your spine, hips, and flanks become free and mobile.

● Wall twist. Stand with your back close to a wall. As you exhale, twist sideways from your hips up to your shoulders, and place your palms on the wall. Remain for 30-60 seconds, breathing regularly. Exhaling, turn to face forward, and repeat on the other side. This relieves tension from your shoulder blades to your hips.

ANAEMIA

In orthodox medicine, anaemia is defined as a lack of normal haemo-globin, the oxygen-carrying pigment in red blood cells. Haemoglobin contains iron, and since red blood cells are continually being made and dying off, the body needs continuing supplies of iron to manufacture more haemoglobin. Thus, for most practical purposes, the kind of anaemia that commonly affects women can be described as being due to lack of iron in the blood. This is known as iron deficiency anaemia.

Anaemia in itself may not be a serious condition. But the associated symptoms of fatigue and depression can affect your whole outlook and ability to cope with life stresses.

Causes of anaemia

The basic problem in most cases of iron-deficiency anaemia is that the body loses more iron, usually in blood, than it obtains from food. The cause of the loss may be heavy periods (see p.114), or pregnancy, where iron is being diverted to the unborn baby.

There are many possible causes of low iron intake. Your diet may lack adequate iron; your dietary iron could be adequate, but your body cannot absorb it properly for some reason; or emotional and higher spiritual features may be involved. Each of these factors is dealt with in turn.

Iron in the diet

Iron is present in a wide range of foods. But a foodstuff's total iron content is not a sure guide. A better indication is its "available iron." This is the amount which can be taken in by a healthy body,

CAUTIONS

There are many types of anaemia and related conditions, some being more serious than others. They include:
- iron deficiency anaemia, as described here,
- pernicious anaemia, involving certain types of poor vitamin B12 absorption, also described here,
- folic-acid deficiency anaemia,
- sickle cell anaemia,
- thalassaemia, and
- haemolytic anaemia.

Before self-treatment, consult a qualified physician for a firm diagnosis of the type of anaemia affecting you.

because not all of the iron in certain foods can be absorbed. The body can only digest and take up iron in the form of soluble salts. If the iron is combined with certain organic compounds which make it insoluble, the body cannot dissolve and digest it.

For example, you might expect that white bread has a lower proportion of total iron than wholegrain brown bread, which it does. But, surprisingly, white bread has more available iron. Similarly, spinach contains a large amount of iron relative to its weight. But it, too, has only a small amount of available iron, because much of its iron is locked in by the chemical oxalic acid.

In general, meats and fish are higher in iron (both total amounts and available iron) than most vegetables and fruits. This puts the vegetarian at a disadvantage when trying to overcome anaemia, although with much attention, this can be corrected (see p.35).

Teas and wholefoods A common substance which affects iron absorption is tea. As explained later, you should avoid all stimulants if you have anaemia, and this applies particularly to tea.

The tannin in tea combines with iron salts in accompanying foods, to make the iron unavailable to the body. (Tea with milk has less effect, since the milk de-activates some of the tannin.)

In a similar way, the bran present in wholefoods contains phytic acid, which combines with iron to make much of it unavailable. (Over time, the body may be able to compensate for such binding effects of phytates.) Thus a particularly devastating combination for the body is to switch suddenly to a vegetarian wholefood diet accompanied by strong, milk-less tea.

FOODS THAT BENEFIT ANAEMIA

Try one or two of the following foods, which should help iron-deficiency anaemia. However, if you feel worse, your anaemia may be due to poor vitamin B12 absorption.

● Brewer's yeast, a heaped 15mls tablespoon, 3 times daily.
● Vitamin E - 50 units daily.
● Wheatgerm.
● Molasses.
● Fenugreek - 1 heaped 5mls teaspoon daily, either in food or as a tea.
● Grape juice.
● A nourishing recipe is 100gms (4ozs) of shrimps and a 5mls teaspoon of black molasses, stewed with a small cup of white wine for 20 minutes.

Vitamin B12 Production of red blood cells requires vitamin B12. The body contains enough B12, chiefly in the liver, to last for a year or two. But it must replenish its supplies from food, so anaemia can be caused by long-term dietary B12 deficiency. This vitamin is present mainly in animal products. It is found in only a few vegetables, when it is made by the natural micro-organisms they carry, and in a few herbs, such as Comfrey (*Symphytum officinale*). So dietary B12 deficiency is a possible risk of a strict, poorly balanced vegetarian diet (see p.36).

Another cause of this type of anaemia is the digestive system's failure to absorb B12, due to conditions affecting the stomach, the intestines, or their natural populations of helpful bacteria. These conditions include gastric or intestinal surgery, for example, as treatment for digestive ulcer. The balance of intestinal bacteria can be upset by recurrent diarrhoea, a very high level of dietary roughage (as used in some "colonic cleansing" programmes), or repeated use of antibiotic drugs.

Iron in the body

Iron is essential for the production of haemoglobin, the red substance in red blood cells. Haemoglobin transports oxygen from the lungs to the tissues of the body. Without iron, the blood becomes "thin," the body tissues lack oxygen, and the characteristic symptoms of anaemia develop. The accompanying discomfort can easily give rise to depression. You feel unable to do anything or to put ideas into action.

In extreme cases, it is difficult to concententrate for any length of time, or to make clear decisions. This is why

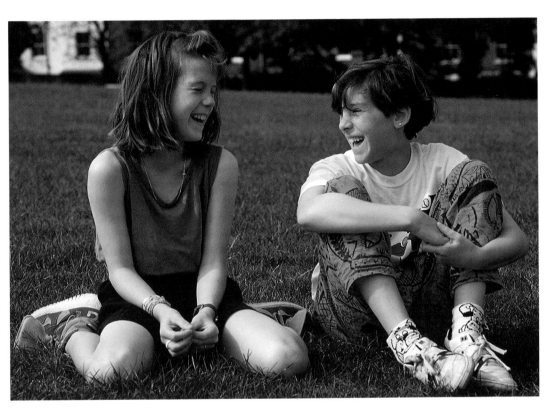

some people with anaemia begin to feel inadequate, feeble, and incapable of tackling everyday life.

Causes in life

Linked closely to the physical problem of not taking in enough available iron, are causes in life itself.

One common factor is a severe illness in childhood, which can have repercussions for the rest of life. In particular, it can unbalance the body so that when you go through a stressful time later in life, anaemia is the likely result.

Another factor involves puberty, one of the "gates" in life (see p.21). If a girl is put under great pressure at this time, or made to feel inadequate, or lacks "space"

Problems during puberty may predispose to anaemia later in life. It is important to allow a girl's individuality to develop as she matures, without repressing her personality, opinions, and ideas.

to develop her own ideas, this can predispose to anaemia later. In particular, it may occur if she has strong opinions but feels unable to express them, for fear of criticism.

Overwork is another factor. The blood nourishes the body with oxygen, which allows thoughts to be translated into action. Therefore a too-active life taxes this function of the blood, and it may also divert your attention from your diet. So a huge workload may help to bring on anaemia.

95

Emotional causes

In anaemia, your muscles are poorly nourished with oxygen, and so become tired and weak. This makes you unable to translate thought into action, which may make you feel inadequate, despairing, frustrated, and discouraged. Yet these emotions, often generated by anaemia, can also be a cause.

If something in your life makes you feel inadequate and lacking the strength to do what you want, this in itself can cause anaemia. Bringing up children, especially, consumes so much time and energy that you may have little of either left for other matters. It may not be possible for you to tackle other things, and so you become frustrated and depressed. These very feelings can contribute to a reduced absorption of dietary iron.

Feelings of inadequacy and depression may be straightforward reactions to a difficult situation, which would affect almost anyone in the same way. But in some cases, the self-view goes deeper. The feelings may have been "built in" to your personality for many years, and present circumstances merely accentuate an attitude formed in childhood.

Such deep-seated feelings can be overcome with the help of counselling, analysis, assertiveness training, and similar techniques.

Societal causes

Anaemia is often linked to factors at a higher level. As explained earlier, one of its main features is difficulty in putting plans into practice, and often the problem is actually at the intellectual level, involving attitudes and ideas.

Our society encourages work and activity, and is built on an attitude of "payment by results." However, in many sectors of society there is a fundamental imbalance.

Women in careers are expected to achieve as much as men, in order to be successful, yet they are often also expected to look after the home and children. Some women react to this attitude with a fierce determination to succeed, both with career and family. This is not always possible. The body and mind can be exhausted, and anaemia may follow.

Patterns of anaemia

There are three main patterns of anaemia: weak energy, low reserves, and poor metabolism. Each has a distinctive course. However, you may find that your particular condition does not fit one pattern exactly, but overlaps with others. This probably means that more than one factor is contributing to your anaemia, which in turn means you should take a combination of steps, including lifestyle changes and career decisions. Combined remedies may also be needed.

General symptoms of anaemia

■ Your face is pale, because there is not enough red haemoglobin in the blood to give your cheeks a healthy pink colour,
■ you become breathless upon exertion, because the blood can take up only low amounts of oxygen from the lungs, and you pant faster to try and absorb more,
■ you experience heart palpitations or "flutters" (tachycardia), because your heart has to pump blood faster in an attempt to distribute enough oxygen,

ARE DIETARY SUPPLEMENTS USEFUL?

Mineral supplements In some cases of anaemia, the body lacks copper, cobalt, and other minerals, besides iron. One way to aid this is to take an all-purpose or combined (compound) mineral supplement, also called a multivitamin multimineral supplement, as available in health food stores. However, if you can, consult a specialist in dietary matters.

Amino acid supplements Amino acids are the building blocks of proteins, the body's chief structural molecules. Taking amino acid supplements can help a generally weak digestion and possibly improve anaemia, although it is wise to consult a dietician or other specialist in this field.

Iron supplements ("iron pills") You can take these in conjunction with natural medicines. To minimize interaction between the medicine and the supplement, leave a gap of at least half an hour between them. However, if iron pills cause severe indigestion, you can take herbal remedies at the same time to overcome this reaction. (See also dietary advice on p.29.)

■ you feel dizzy, because not enough oxygen reaches your brain, and you are generally tired and dispirited.

General guidance on treatment

Treatment of anaemia is much more successful if you can establish the cause. In particular, talk to someone about your condition, and about your problems and the way you feel. A family practitioner, or perhaps a close friend, may see matters more clearly.

Some homeopathic and herbal remedies may make you feel more tired at first, because of their relaxing effects. You must accept this, for it is true that anaemia is a "weak" disease, and the body needs rest to build up strength.

Diet In addition to major dietary guidelines, try the following:
● Avoid stimulants such as tea and coffee - no more than one cup daily. The problem of anaemia is related to your body not responding to your will. Stimulants temporarily increase the will's grip on the body, so it seems easier to force yourself onward. But this masks the real trouble, and when the stimulants wear off, the situation worsens.

You may find it extremely difficult to give up these stimulants, since they are truly addictive drugs. If so, consult a practitioner of natural medicine. She or he can give support and suggest ways of obtaining the energy you need, so that you can gradually wean yourself from the drugs.
● Avoid alcohol, especially if you suffer from the "lack of cool" pattern of anaemia. Limit yourself to two glasses of wine or its equivalent (two standard units or "shots" of alcohol) each week.
● Avoid sugar and high-sugar foods. They may give you a temporary lift of

energy, but this "rush" is soon followed by a corresponding drop.

● Eat plenty of good-quality food which has high vitality, which means it has not been overcooked, processed, or frozen.

● Eat organic foods.

● Ensure that your food contains sufficient high-quality protein, in addition to sufficient iron.

● If you take iron supplements, make sure the iron is in a form that your body can absorb. Some "iron pills," for example those containing ferrous sulphate, can be hard to digest. They may upset your body so much that you lose more iron (through heavy periods and in other ways) and absorb less iron, due to a weakened digestion.

Homeopathy Anaemia responds particularly well to the "constitutional" type of homeopathic prescribing (see p.56). However, this is difficult to do in the home, so consult a practitioner if you feel this treatment may benefit you.

General homeopathic remedies for anaemia include China, especially when there has been great loss of blood, and also Ferr. met. or Selenium.

"Weak energy" pattern

In this pattern, your overall energy (see p.14) has become low, often because of factors such as too much work, disturbed sleep, and lack of support from others. If you have a blood test, you may find that besides lack of iron, you are also low on minerals, vitamins, amino acids, and other blood components. This is reflected in a loss of energy, depressed emotions, and weak willpower.

Typical symptoms, in addition to the general ones listed on p.96, are:

■ your tongue is pale and perhaps coated with "fur," and your eyes are dull, distant, and lifeless,

■ your appetite is poor,

■ you lack interests, pursuits, or hobbies in life,

■ you may be prone to tears,

■ you need extra sleep , and

■ your pulse rate is unusually slow when sitting or lying.

"Lack of cool" pattern

Your reserves of cool, calm energy are depleted, as is your blood energy (this is explained on pp.14-17). One cause is a strong will driving the body too hard.

This may originate from leading an exceptionally interesting and creative life, being in the centre of activity. More often, it comes from restlessness and discontent. You may see your life as dull and colourless, and this makes you agitated and restless - largely futile feelings that use up valuable energy. When you have time to sit still and reflect, you lack the cool, calm energy to do so. Discontent rises up and stimulates further frantic activity, that dissipates energy which should otherwise be available for translating rational thoughts into actions.

Typical symptoms, in addition to the general ones for anaemia, are:

■ a pale face, but pink or red cheeks,

■ a "glittery" look in your eyes, and dark rings round them,

■ you are generally restless, with a highly stimulated mind in which one idea soon crowds out another,

■ you have difficulty going to sleep,

■ you experience night sweats and perhaps daytime "flushes," and

■ your pulse is rapid and "thready."

TREATMENT FOR WEAK ENERGY PATTERN OF ANAEMIA

Aims of treatment

Treatment is directed at changing the balance of your life, by reducing demands so that you can save energy. To make such changes, you need to organize help in your daily life, and so free time for yourself. As with all forms of anaemia, try to find the cause, and assess your diet and ways of improving its available iron content.

Herbs

Note: See p.38 for doses and cautions for herbs.
● Gentian (*Gentiana lutea*), Berberis (*Berberis vulgaris*), Licorice (*Glycyrrhiza glabra*), and Wild yam (*Dioscorea villosa*). Standard dose (40 drops of mixed tincture), 3 times daily in water. Gentian is a tonic for the stomach and the whole system; Berberis is a tonic to the stomach and improves assimilation, and also helps to move the energy. Licorice increases energy, while Wild yam helps to balance the female hormones.
● If you are extremely weak, add Ginseng (*Panax ginseng*), 600mgs per day.
● Other herbs of use are Nettles (*Urtica dioica*) and White poplar (*Populus tremuloides*).

Homeopathy

Note: See p.54 for doses and cautions for homeopathic remedies.
  Take the remedy 3 times daily for 2-3 months. Start with 6X potency. If there has been no change after 2 weeks, select another remedy. If the remedy works at first, then the effects wear off, increase the potency, under the guidance of a homeopath.
● If you feel anxious and lack support - Calc. carb.
● If you have difficulty in showing or even feeling affection, and experience dragging sensations in the pelvis - Sepia.
● If you are generally nervous and sensitive, and prone to chills - Ars. alb.
● Other remedies include Causticum and Carbo veg.

Exercises

Note: See p.70 for details of exercise routines.
● Weak routine, slowly graduating to Easy routine.

If, in addition, your tongue has a cracked surface and a red tip, this may be a sign of anaemia caused by lack of vitamin B12 (see p.94).

General advice Foremost is the need to bring calm and serenity into your life. You may find this awkward at first, since you may think that a calmer life means less action and enjoyment. In fact, you may experience these sensations during the first few weeks of slowing down. But then you should find that life gradually becomes richer, and fuller.

Imagine the analogy of colour. In a hectic lifestyle, the interesting parts have gaudy primary hues, rather like a child's plastic toys; the rest of life takes on drab tones.

When you first slow down, the drab backdrop remains, but the primary colours - life's "fun" - fade. However, after a few weeks, you become accustomed to life's new level of colours. With a few overpoweringly bright items gone, the whole landscape is full of so many different hues, which you now have time to study and savour.

"Poor metabolism" pattern

In this pattern, you may not place excessive demands on your body and its energy, but your overall production of energy has become blocked and obstructed. The cause may be a physical difficulty, or a residue from an illness such as hepatitis, glandular fever, or recurrent severe diarrhoea. Or there may be an emotional basis, for example, inability to accept a change in your life, or holding onto a grudge or insult. Another possibility could involve rela-

---

TREATMENT FOR LACK OF COOL PATTERN OF ANAEMIA

As with all forms of anaemia, try to find the cause, and assess your diet and ways of improving its available iron content.

Herbs

Note: See p.38 for doses and cautions for herbs.
   Take the standard dose, 3 times daily.
● Lady's slipper (*Cypripedium pubescens*), Beth root (*Trillium pendulum*), Water lily (*Nymphaea alba*), and Yarrow (*Achillea millefolium*). Lady's slipper calms; Beth root and Water lily strengthen the lower part of the body, helping to draw energy down; while Yarrow is a balancing tonic that assists control of flushes and heat.
● If you have insomnia, add Passion flower (*Passiflora incarnata*) or Valerian (*Valeriana officinalis*).

Homeopathy

Note: See p.54 for doses and cautions for homeopathic remedies.
   Take the remedy 3 times daily for 2-3 months. Start with 6X potency. If there has been no change after 2 weeks, select another remedy. If the remedy works at first, then the effects wear off, increase the potency under the guidance of a homeopath.
● If you have a great thirst for cold water, and you are easily startled - Phosphorus.
● If you twitch and "start" on going to sleep, and you desire alcohol - Lachesis.
● If you have a tendency to heat and inflammations, and need stimulants - Ferr. phos.
● If you are resentful and hold long-standing grudges - Nit. ac.

Exercises

Note: See p.70 for details of exercise routines.
● Easy routine.
● Crawl around a well-carpeted floor for 5-10 minutes daily. Try to make your movements lithe and purposeful.

crawling

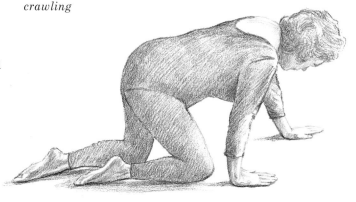

tionships, both with other adults and in your family. You may experience very powerful feelings, but no opportunity presents to express them. All these factors interfere with your normal flow of energy, leaving insufficient supplies for the everyday things in your life.

Symptoms Typical symptoms, in addition to the general ones for anaemia, include:
■ you may be overweight,
■ your complexion is pasty,
■ there is a coat on your tongue,
■ you have an irregular appetite, eating lots and then little, and you crave sweet foods,
■ your digestion is generally poor, and you suffer diarrhoea, and also fluid retention leading to puffiness around the face and ankles,
■ your pulse is weak, deep, and difficult to find, and
■ you appear jovial on the outside, but you are gloomy or angry within.

From this description of the patterns of anaemia, and the way the life causes interact, it can be seen that this is sometimes not an easy condition to cure. You may have to coordinate changes in several areas, including your commitments to family and work, your diet and lifestyle, and your reserves of energy and your energy circulation.

The simple orthodox medical blood test for anaemia, which detects low levels of healthy haemoglobin, is therefore only the tip of the matter. It is worth emphasizing that diet is an especially important factor, and there are many specialist publications now available in this area (see p.186).

In addition, review your ability to express your deeply-held emotions and feelings, which may be kept below the surface by your family, professional, or social situation.

TREATMENT FOR POOR METABOLISM PATTERN OF ANAEMIA

Aims of treatment

In this pattern, physical and emotional problems usually combine, so act on both. As with all forms of anaemia, try to establish the cause. On the physical level, adjust the balance of your body so that it can digest food fully and absorb the iron. On the emotional level, try to resolve any grievance or grudge, in order to redirect the emotional energy that is being consumed in supporting negative emotions.

Diet

Assess your diet and improve its available iron content.

Herbs

Note: See p.38 for doses and cautions for herbs.

● Golden seal (*Hydrastis canadensis*), Black root (*Leptandra virginica*), Fringe tree (*Chionanthus virginica*), and Agrimony (*Agrimonia eupatorium*). Golden seal is a tonic and stimulates the digestion, helping to clear mucus (phlegm). Black root also tonifies, especially the liver. Fringe tree increases the

Continued on next page

Continued from previous page

flow of bile, and Agrimony is a stimulant and general tonic.
● If you have constipation, add Cascara (*Rhamnus purshiana*).

Homeopathy

Note: See p.54 for doses and cautions for homeopathic remedies.
Take the remedy 3 times daily for 2-3 months. Start with 6X potency. If there has been no change after 2 weeks, select another remedy. If the remedy works at first, then the effects wear off, increase the potency under the guidance of a homeopath.
● If you tend to burst into tears, and you have green discharges - Pulsatilla.
● If you feel generally irritable, with watery nasal discharge - Nat. mur.
● If you fear being alone, and you suffer constipation with a swollen lower abdomen - Lycopodium.
● Other remedies to consider are Apis mel., Chamomilla, Cyclamen, Graphites, Helonias, Mercurius, and Silica.

Exercises

Note: See p.54 for details of exercise routines.
● Alternate between the Strong and Dynamic routines, one daily.
● Do Neck stand and Plough daily, except during your period, when you should substitute:
● Hum dum. Stand relaxed, with your palms resting on slightly bent knees. Keep your neck in line with the rest of your spine. Slowly twist your neck to the left, saying "Hum," then to the right as you say "Dum." Continue for 2-3 minutes in an easy rhythm. Then stand up straight and lean back, resting your hands lightly on your buttocks, looking slightly up. Repeat the neck twists as you say "Hum, Dum" again, for 2-3 minutes. This subtle exercise greatly benefits the metabolism, via the thyroid gland in the neck, giving you a restful feeling.

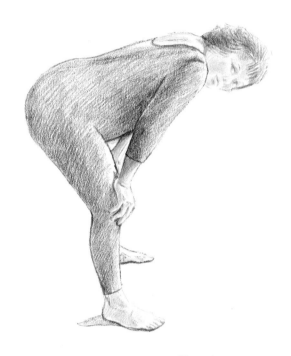

Hum dum

VAGINAL DISCHARGE AND ITCHING

A small amount of vaginal discharge is not unusual, especially around ovulation (see p.89), and just before and after the period. However, some women suffer from a continuous and heavy discharge. Besides being unpleasant and embarrassing, this may also encourage germs and infection. In some cases, the discharge gives rise to intense itching.

Causes

In natural medicine, there are two main patterns of vaginal discharge: "excess mucus" and "weak." The first is a manifestation of accumulated mucus (phlegm) in the body. The second is due to weakness in the lower part of the body, which gives rise to poor circulation of fluids. It is said that the fluids go the "wrong way," and instead of being excreted by the kidneys, they collect in the lower body, and find the easiest way out.

Sexual factors There may be a connection between over-production of mucus and a certain mental state. A mind that rejects the body's physical functions as degrading or unclean may become separated from the physical body because of deeply-hidden feelings of uncleanliness and shame concerning sex.

Many people have ambivalent attitudes about sex. They may approve of it, and indeed view it as one of life's main purposes. Yet they are very reserved and secretive about it. Sex is natural, and the rational mind emphasizes this. However, the broad spectrum of feelings on the subject may cause the mind to become partially separated from the physical body's sexual functions. If you have feelings of uncleanliness about sexual matters, counselling or psychotherapy can be recommended. A natural treatment which may assist is the Bach flower remedy Crab apple (see p.186).

"Weak" pattern

Symptoms This general pattern is described on p.98. In addition:
■ the discharge is thin and watery, and worse when you are exhausted,
■ you are generally tired, with a pale face and slight anaemia,
■ you have backaches, especially when tired, and you need to sit down a lot,
■ you suffer bad feelings after the period, and
■ there is a dragging sensation in your lower abdomen.

Natural remedies can be of great assistance. You may need to cut back on your daily schedule, and the remedies should help you to see the best way of doing this, as explained for period problems (see p.106).

DANGER SIGNS

Vaginal discharge and/or itching may be due to a condition that could, if untreated, lead to more serious problems. Consult a qualified practitioner of either orthodox or natural medicine for a diagnosis, before you begin self-treatment, especially if:
■ you suspect a sexually-transmitted disease is causing the trouble,
■ you have additional symptoms, such as swollen glands, skin rash, or high fever, or
■ the problem does not clear up after about three months, or suddenly becomes more severe.

"Excess mucus" pattern

Symptoms The following symptoms and signs typically occur:
■ the discharge tends to be rather thick and white or yellow,
■ you may have genital itching, and
■ you may develop an infection, which shows as a copious, thick, yellow discharge, and
■ you may also have other signs of over-production of mucus, including greasy hair, a shiny nose, and possibly a blocked nose, postnasal drip, or phlegm collecting in the throat.

General advice The symptoms of mucus discharge are nearly always related to a general imbalance in the body, so they respond well to changes which reduce the level of mucus in the whole system. In particular, avoid mucus-producing foods such as milk, cheese, peanuts, and sugary foods. Try to cut down on alcohol. Eat more mucus-lowering foods, such as garlic, onion, watercress, and spices like cardamon and mustard.

In some women, the excess mucus is related to a mild allergy, either to gluten (see p.34), or to foods made with yeasts, such as breads and beers.

TREATMENT FOR WEAK PATTERN OF VAGINAL DISCHARGE

Herbs

Note: See p.38 for doses and cautions for herbs.
● Beth root (*Trillium pendulum*), False unicorn root (*Chamaelirium luteum*), White poplar (*Populus tremuloides*), and Cranesbill (*Geranium maculatum*).
● An alternative to Cranesbill is Tormentil (*Potentilla tormentilla*).

Take the herbs for at least three months, especially the first two, which strengthen the pelvic area.

Homeopathy

Note: See p.54 for doses and cautions for homeopathic remedies.
● If you have difficulty expressing your feelings, a dragging sensation in your lower abdomen, and the discharge is yellow or green, perhaps with itching - Sepia.
● If you tend to catch colds, and the discharge is watery - Nat. mur.
● If you have "hot" feelings, especially in the head, and you suffer nasal mucus and weakness - Calc. carb.
● If you feel chilly a lot of the time, and you are nervous and frightened - Ars. alb.

Exercises

Note: See p.70 for details of exercise routines.
● Easy or Weak routine.
● Moth (see p.6). Lie on your front, arms pointing back. Exhaling, raise your legs, arms, and chest off the floor. Hold this position for 30-60 seconds, exhale, and lower yourself back to the floor. This exercise invigoratingly contracts your sacrum.
● Pelvic energizer. Try it lying on your back, knees bent. Learn it in three phases. First, become aware of the tough muscular ring of your anal sphincter. Try to raise and lower it at will, holding it up and tight for 3-4 seconds at a time. Notice a tingling sensation in the pelvic area. Second, spread this ability to your whole pelvic floor, contracting and relaxing it. Third, become aware of the inner anal sphincter just above the outer one. Raise and lower both of these as you contract and relax your whole lower abdomen, bringing energy to the area.

TREATMENT FOR EXCESS MUCUS PATTERN OF VAGINAL DISCHARGE

Herbs

Note: See p.38 for doses and cautions for herbs.
● Golden seal (*Hydrastis canadensis*), Balmony (*Celone glabra*), and Cranesbill (*Geranium maculatum*). Golden seal and Balmony both assist in reducing mucus, and both have a special effect on the reproductive system. Cranesbill is generally drying.

When you first take Golden seal and Balmony, there may be an increase in mucus for the first week or so. Then it and the discharge should gradually reduce. Continue taking the herbs for a month after the discharge has gone.
● If you also have a strong sexual urge - add Water lily (*Nymphaea alba*) to the above prescription.
● If the discharge is a yellow-green - add St John's wort (*Hypericum perfoliatum*).

Homeopathy

Note: See p.54 for doses and cautions for homeopathic remedies.
● If you feel emotionally bruised, your leg glands are swollen, and you have sensations of numbness - Conium.
● If the discharge is greenish - Merc. sol.

● If the discharge is creamy - Pulsatilla.
● If the discharge is offensive and burning - Nit. ac.
● If the discharge causes itching - Graphites.
● If the discharge is thick and yellow, and causes itching - Sulphur.
● If the discharge causes stinging sensations - Kreasotum.

Exercises

Note: See p.70 for details of exercise routines.
● Dynamic routine.
● Camel. Kneel, with your trunk and thighs vertical. Exhaling, lean back and place your hands on your feet behind you. Tilting your head back, move your pelvis forward as far as you can.
● Bellows breathing. Sit comfortably and breathe slowly for 3 minutes. After a long, slow inhalation, exhale fast and forcefully. Repeat 10-15 times. You may well feel slightly dizzy or experience strange muscular sensations; this is normal. Finally, begin to breathe slowly and restfully again, feeling aware and refreshed.

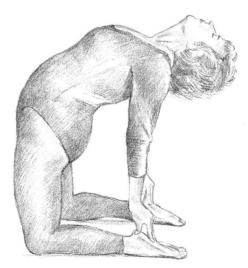

Camel

PERIOD PAINS

Pain during the period is so common and widespread that many women consider it normal. The pain can be so severe that they are incapacitated for several days each month. In most cases, the condition is "functional" (see p.12). There is no obvious physical or physiological abnormality, and so it cannot really be helped by orthodox medicine - except possibly by hormonal or anti-inflammatory pills. But many women instinctively reject this solution. Such functional problems usually respond well to natural medicine.

Causes

Physically, period pain is due to spasms, cramps or aches in the muscle tissues of your uterus (womb) and cervix (neck of the womb), and in related muscular parts such as your lower back and down into your upper legs. Orthodox medicine has shown that these spasms may be related to hormonal or dietary imbalance; the corresponding treatment is to prescribe anti-inflammatory, hormonal or diet supplement pills (such as extra calcium).

But hormonal imbalance is usually just one aspect of a much wider pattern of imbalance. To provide a lasting cure, rather than temporary alleviation of

CAUTION

Period pains may be severe and even incapacitating, but they rarely signify a life-threatening condition. If you treat yourself with natural medicines, but do not improve after three months, visit an orthodox medical practitioner for advice.

symptoms, you need to consider your whole condition. This means identifying which of the four common patterns of period pain affects you.

"Fatigue" pattern

On the physical level, the period pain is mainly due to some kind of tiredness or weakness. Just as your leg muscles ache after unaccustomed heavy work or when you are generally tired, so the uterine muscles ache when they are exhausted, or if they are made to work when the whole body is tired.

The causes of fatigue are many. For effective treatment, try to distinguish whether the fatigue is localized in your uterus, or whether it is an overall body condition. Common causes include:

■ Too much work, when you always have too many tasks and activities, which eventually deplete your whole energy. This may happen at work, with a very demanding job, or in the home, if you have several children and a house to run - or both. The effort involved may be just too great.

■ Over-stimulation, when all your energy is directed into an excessively stimulated life; when your period comes, you lack sufficient energy to cope.

■ Anaemia (see p.93), when there is insufficient healthy blood to nourish the uterine muscles in their activity.

■ Lack of time to recover after childbirth, which can be very exhausting, especially for the energy in the uterus.

Emotional level Symptoms of the fatigue type of period pain are likely if your emotional energy (see p.14) is weak. This weakening often occurs after an emotionally draining time, such as when

TREATMENT FOR FATIGUE PATTERN OF PERIOD PAINS

Natural medicine can be very helpful in treating this condition, but do not expect miracles. Herbs and homeopathic remedies may supply you with more energy, but they cannot replace human support, nor can they provide enough energy for an over-ambitious schedule.

Herbs

Note: See p.38 for doses and cautions for herbs.
• Tonic herbs include Beth root (*Trillium pendulum*), False unicorn root (*Chamaelirium luteum*), True unicorn root (*Aletris farinosa*), Stone root (*Collinsonia canadensis*), Rhatany root (*Krameria triandra*), and Ginseng (*Panax ginseng*).
  Select 2-3 of these tonic herbs, and combine with a moving herb, such as White poplar (*Populus tremuloides*) or Gentian (*Gentiana lutea*). Do not take the tonics on their own, since they may cause tightening and increase the cramps slightly.
  After 1-2 weeks, you should notice an improvement, but it may take a year or more to recover if your various body systems have become very depleted of energy.

• Home prescription - Beth root, False unicorn root, and White poplar.

Homeopathy

Note: See p.54 for doses and cautions for homeopathic remedies.
• If you feel despair and find it difficult to show affection, and you have a dragging sensation in your lower abdomen - Sepia.
• If you sense a lack of support, and you suffer from nasal mucus and difficulty digesting milk - Calc. carb.
• If your tiredness comes from mental work, and you have a tendency to headaches and nerve pains - Actea racemosa.

Exercises

Note: See p.70 for details of exercise routines.
• Weak routine, plus:

Pelvic balancer

• Pelvic balancer. Lie down with fingers interlocked behind your head, knees bent, soles flat on the floor. Lower one knee sideways to the floor. Inhale deeply, then exhale as you raise your hips off the floor as high as you can; hold for a few seconds; lower them again with an exhalation. Repeat several times. Repeat the pattern with the other knee lowered instead. Then repeat again, on the easier side. This exercise stretches away tiredness in the lower organs and restores equilibrium to the two sides of your pelvis.

Food supplements

If you feel very tired and depleted, consider taking vitamin, mineral, and amino acid supplements.

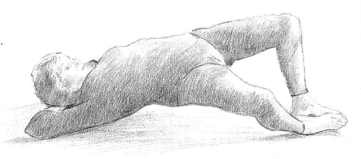

nursing a sick child, or coping with a difficult parent. Your physical body may not show signs of fatigue, but you no longer have the desire to go out and face the world; these feelings are further aggravated by your period.

Another cause at the emotional level is a "distaste" for the period itself (see p.114). You may think that there is something "not quite right" about the period, perhaps as a result of the attitudes of parents or friends during your upbringing. This can bring on a tendency to withdraw energy from the uterus throughout the entire cycle. As a result, when your period starts, your uterine muscles lack the energy to function well.

Symptoms Typical symptoms for the fatigue pattern of period pain include:
■ pain that starts after your period, and that continues for a few days when the period stops,
■ the pain is more of a dull ache, with "bearing-down" sensations, and is worse when you are generally tired,
■ backache and fatigue, which get worse as the period continues, and
■ your face is pale, and you feel "washed out" afterward.

There may be additional symptoms linked to anaemia (p.96), or to a general shortage of creative energy (see p.18).

"Blockage" pattern

The physical basis of the blockage pattern is poor liver function. Hormones are metabolized in the liver, and any problem there may lead to hormonal imbalance. At the physical level, causes include an over-rich diet, too much coffee or alcohol or chocolate, and lack of physical exercise, all of which are

---

FIRST AID FOR PERIOD PAINS

If you commonly suffer sudden, excruciating menstrual cramps, keep one of these remedies with you at all times, at home, at work, and in the car.
● Homeopathic Caulophyllum at 6X potency. Take 2 small pills dissolved under the tongue, every 15 minutes.
● Herbal Cramp bark (*Viburnum opulus*) as mother tincture. Take 5 drops in a little warm water.

---

detrimental to your liver. The contraceptive pill and other medicinal drugs are also dealt with by the liver.

You may experience the blockage in the form of headaches, mild indigestion, overweight, and general irritability. When your period is due, the activity of the uterus is also blocked, and the symptoms are aggravated.

Emotional level If you are often frustrated or angry, and bottle up these feelings, the normal circulation of energy is obstructed. A woman living in a "man's world" can also develop this pattern, especially when she has to fight for position and respect.

A more subtle cause of blockage on the emotional level comes from the habit of trying too hard. Our society places so much emphasis on material results, and so little on the qualities of stillness and warmth, that many women (and men) feel their worth is measured by daily achievements. This creates a constant pressure to get on and succeed, which leads to continual pushing of the body's energy circulation. You may experience this as an extended state of general body

TREATMENT FOR BLOCKAGE PATTERN OF PERIOD PAINS

Herbs

Note: See p.38 for doses and cautions for herbs.

● Chamomile (*Matricaria chamomilla*) is a mild uterine relaxant, and also an easily obtainable herb.

Relaxants that work specifically on the uterus are Blue cohosh (*Caulophyllum thalactroides*), Cramp bark (*Viburnum opulus*), and Catmint (*Nepeta cataria*).

● Valerian (*Valeriana officinalis*) is a general relaxant.

● Home prescription - Blue cohosh, Catmint, and Valerian.

Take the herbs for 10-14 days before the expected date of your period (ideally from ovulation, if you know its date).

Homeopathy

Note: See p.54 for doses and cautions for homeopathic remedies.

● If you have an excitable temperament, with thick nasal mucus, and bad feelings in damp weather - Gelsemium.

● If you are often irritated and angry, and suffer shooting pains in the hips which improve when you move about - Chamomilla.

● If you tend to burst into tears, and have green discharges from the nose and elsewhere - Pulsatilla.

● If the pain starts with the period itself, there is strong bleeding with clots, and you feel grudging - Ignatia.

● If the pain is colicky and cramping, starts a day or two before the period, and is worse at night, but improves with the blood flow - Mag. phos.

● If the pain has a shooting nature - Cimicifuga.

Take one of the above remedies for 8-10 days before your period starts, or as a constitutional remedy in high potencies before the period.

Exercises

Note: See p.70 for details of exercise routines.

● Dynamic routine, plus:

● Twist and bend. Sit comfortably. Interlock your fingers just above your head. As you exhale, bend your trunk to one side. Inhale as your straighten. Repeat to the other side. Then as you exhale, twist your trunk to one side while staying vertical, as far as you can go. Inhale as you face the front, and repeat the twist to the other side. Repeat these four actions 10-20 times to free your trunk of its "straitjacket."

Twist and bend

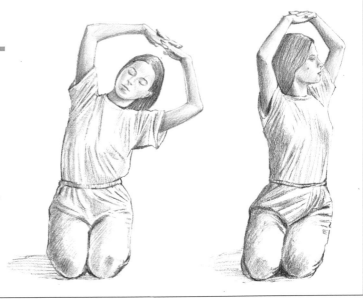

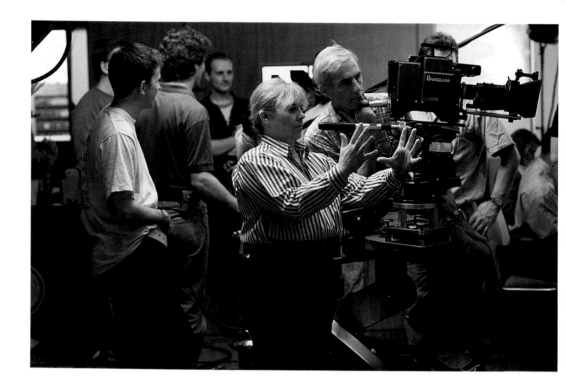

The pressures of demanding work can feed through the emotional and mental levels, to the basic physical level, causing period pain.

tension; when your period comes, it may bring on spasms or cramps in the muscles of the uterus.

Symptoms Typical symptoms of the blockage pattern of period pain include:
■ a cramping pain, which is often relieved after the first day or two,
■ your breasts and abdomen are swollen and tender beforehand, and
■ you are irritable before the period, but relieved when it has started.
  Additional symptoms include headache, craving for sweet foods, a furry tongue, and exhaustion in the morning yet feeling wide awake at night.

"Cold" pattern

On the physical level, the cold pattern of period pain is chiefly due to getting too cold. The body is especially vulnerable to chills during the menstrual period. You may also be vulnerable just after lovemaking, when the uterus is receptive to the aggressive forces of nature. If the cause really is physical, the cold usually

CAUTION

Symptoms involving heavy uterine bleeding may have an underlying physical cause, such as uterine fibroids. Before you start treatment, consult a qualified practitioner.

has a clear origin. You may be able to trace it back to an event such as a sudden chilly wind, when you were unprepared. The pain is caused by cramps in the uterine muscles, in the way that any muscle can tense and tighten in cold weather.

In Western society, where people are less exposed to the physical elements, the cause of the cold pattern is often found at the emotional or spiritual level. It may be associated with a "cold" feeling towards sexual matters, or repulsion and "shivers" at the thought of sexual activity. Another possibility is too much mental work, which by nature is cold and calculating. Or the cold pattern may be due to insufficient spiritual energy nour-

TREATMENT FOR COLD PATTERN OF PERIOD PAINS

Treatment is most likely to succeed if the cause is truly physical. Take the remedies for about 10 days before your period starts.

Herbs

Note: See p.38 for doses and cautions for herbs.
• Yarrow (*Achillea mille-folium*), Ginger (*Zingiber officinale*), and Cramp bark (*Viburnum opulus*). To a cup of warm water, add a 5mls teaspoon of infusion of dried Yarrow, a little fresh grated Ginger, and 10 drops of tincture of Cramp bark. Sip 1 cup 3 times daily before the period, and every 2 hours when the pain is present. Add a teaspoon of molasses to the mixture, if available.

External remedies

You can apply the above herbs externally at the time of menstruation. Pour a teaspoon of tincture onto the absorbent side of a waterproof dressing and place it on the skin over the painful area. Replace the dressing 3-4 times daily.

Homeopathy

Note: See p.54 for doses and cautions for homeopathic remedies.
• If you are fearful but without perspiration, and the chills are severe and of recent origin (such as catching cold or eating bad food) - Aconite.
• If your chills are less severe but last longer, and you tend to nervousness or fear with perspiration - Ars. alb. (The fear is not so severe as with Aconite, being more of a persistent anxiety.)
• If your cramping pains resemble abdominal flatulence - Colocynth.
• If the pains are accompanied by diarrhoea and a cold, sweaty forehead, and you feel faint to the point of collapse - Veratrum album.
   Take the remedies when the pain appears, or if the problem should recur, try constitutional potencies as described on p.56.

Exercises

Note: See p.70 for details of exercise routines.
• The Great pull. Sit on the floor with your legs straight in front. Bend one knee outward, placing its foot against the opposite thigh. Lean forward and grasp the toes of the straight leg. Tuck your chin into your breastbone. Squeeze your lower belly against your spine as you gaze at your toes, breathing deeply and rhythmically. Feel the welcome flow of energy into your lower abdomen, focusing onto the uterus. Remain for 30-60 seconds, exhale slowly as you relax and return to the starting position, and repeat the Great pull on the other side.

ishing the creative system (see p.18). This may happen if your creative energy lacks an outlet or is suppressed. For example, a mother who is very jealous of her daughter can prevent her "escaping" from the role of being a child and developing her full creative powers. Or you may have a powerful need for creative expression, but your daily routine and family commitments do not allow this.

Symptoms Typical symptoms of the cold pattern of period pain include:
■ the period is scanty and may be late,

TREATMENT FOR "FULL HEAT" HOT PATTERN OF PERIOD PAINS

This pattern is relatively easy to cure - if you can identify the source of the heat. Avoid hot-type foods (see p.33); since many are meats, consider becoming a vegetarian. However, ensure adequate intake of vitamin B12 to counteract anaemia (see p.93).

Herbs

Note: See p.38 for doses and cautions for herbs.
● Shepherd's purse (*Capsella bursa-pastoris*), Marigold petals (*Calendula officinalis*), and Sage (*Salvia officinalis*). Shepherd's purse regulates the blood flow, Marigold clears heat from the body, and the gentle tonic Sage balances the prescription.

Homeopathy

Note: See p.54 for doses and cautions for homeopathic remedies.
● If the pain is worse in the morning, and you feel hypersensitive, with general heat through your body, and a tendency to headaches - Belladonna.
● If you are irritable or jealous, and suffer urine retention with stinging sensations - Apis mel.
● If you suffer great pain, and your vagina and vulva are very tender - Coffea.
● If your pain is mainly around the base of your back, and you are very stressed - Nux vomica.

Exercises

Note: See p.70 for details of exercise routines.
● Strong routine. Include

Bow

Pelvic balancer (see p.107) and Brandysnap breathing (see p.18). Also:
● Bow, to let heat disperse from your lower abdomen. Lie on your front, bend your knees and grasp your ankles. Keeping your knees together, exhale and raise your thighs and chest from the floor, to balance on your navel area. Separate your knees as you raise yourself higher for a few seconds, then bring knees back together and remain for 30-60 seconds. Exhale as you slowly relax and gently release your ankles.

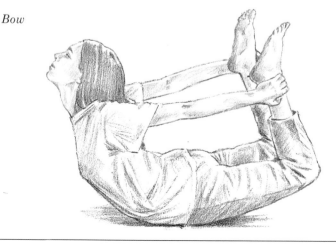

- the pain is so severe and cramping that you may double up in agony, and
- you feel chilly or cold, and gain relief from a hot water bottle applied to the lower abdomen.

Often the whole character and appearance is affected, with signs such as feeling cold, pale face and lips, and a reserved personality.

"Hot" pattern

On the physical level, this pattern occurs when the whole body becomes too warm. A contributing factor is hot-type foods (see p.33). Your emotional state is also important, since it determines many of the symptoms. Consider if you identify with one of these two characteristic emotional types.

You may be strong, vigorous and energetic, with no difficulty in expressing your feelings. However the feelings are generally very stormy, and you are often frustrated and red-faced. The Chinese call this "full heat."

The second emotional type is known to the Chinese as "empty heat." You are generally tense, and find it difficult to express your feelings, which you are prone to keep bottled up. These emotional aspects are reflected physically by heat accumulating in the uterus. Although you feel hot inside, your hands and feet are cold.

Symptoms For the "full heat" type of period pains:
- your face is flushed and red,
- your period may be early and heavy,
- you tend to bleed easily when cut or bruised, as with nosebleeds, and
- you feel generally hot and energetic.

In the "empty heat" pattern the symptoms are very similar to those for the "lack of cool" pattern of anaemia (see p.98), except that:
- only your cheeks are red,
- you have heavy menstrual bleeding,
- your feet feel cold to the touch, and
- your body is generally tense and your muscles are "tight."

TREATMENT FOR "EMPTY HEAT" HOT PATTERN OF PERIOD PAINS

This pattern is difficult to cure, and requires work at the emotional level. The remedies here can help, but you are advised to consult a practitioner of natural medicine, for help with expressing emotions and overcommitment.

Exercises

See "Full heat" pattern, opposite.

Herbs

Note: See p.38 for doses and cautions for herbs.
- Lady's slipper (*Cypripedium pubescens*), Passion flower (*Passiflora incarnata*), and Black cohosh (*Cimicifuga racemosa*). These relaxing herbs can help you to slow down and sleep.
- Another helpful herb is Brazilian ginseng (*Pfaffia paniculata*), available from many health shops.

Homeopathy

Note: See p.54 for doses and cautions for homeopathic remedies.
- If you startle easily and feel insecure - Phosphorus.
- If you have a tendency to spots, and to compulsions such as endless talking, or gambling - Lachesis.

HEAVY PERIODS

The blood lost during the period is due to breakdown and shedding of the lining of the uterus (womb). In some cases, more blood is lost than is necessary for this process, and the period is said to be "heavy." In mild cases this can lead to embarrassment, discomfort, and fatigue. In severe cases it can bring on anaemia (see p.93), or even require first aid, as a blood transfusion.

When your periods continue to be heavy over a long time, and the repeated loss of blood represents a significant threat to health, orthodox forms of treatment include hysterectomy (see p.174) or endometrial ablation. Hysterectomy is often advised if you are certain you no longer wish to have children, or if you are approaching the menopause. However, there may well be no need for surgery. Natural remedies are usually very effective in regulating abnormally heavy periods (provided the problem is "functional," as described below, and without complications). To choose the correct remedy, do not view the symptoms in isolation, but consider the many factors that influence your life.

There are four main patterns of heavy menstrual bleeding. However, in practice there is overlap, so you may wish to select remedies for more than one.

"Weak" pattern

The weak pattern occurs because your body's energy, particularly in the uterus, has become very low. Its main causes are those which drain energy - overwork, stressful situations, too many demands on time, too much physical work, and lack of sleep.

At the emotional level, an important factor is spending too much time and

CAUTIONS

Several serious health problems can cause heavy periods, such as:
- uterine fibroids,
- endometriosis,
- a blood-clotting disorder,
- increased blood pressure,
- cervical erosion, and
- cancer of the cervix or uterus.

Before you start self-treatment, consult a qualified practitioner of natural or othodox medicine.

effort providing emotional support for others, such as partners, parents, and children. This causes a net outflow of energy. If you are overtaxed in this way, or feel unsupported by those around, energy may drain away.

At higher levels, many of the causes of anaemia can reduce your available energy. In particular, negative feelings about menstruation and sexual matters may lower the energy in the uterus. This can produce a "vicious circle." Excessive bleeding is due to lack of energy and negative experiences with periods, but it further lowers uterine energy, so that you dread the next period even more.

Symptoms The following features characterize the weak pattern:
- your menstrual bleeding is heavy and debilitating,
- it is worse when you are tired, and better if you lie down and rest,
- it is also helped by warmth, such as a hot water bottle on the area,
- the blood is bright red, or pale red if you have anaemia,
- periods are regular or slightly late,

114

■ if you have period pain, it tends to be more of an ache, and worse toward the end of the period, and
■ you may have other signs such as a pale face with no "glow," lacklustre hair, and tired, dull eyes.

"Lack of cool" pattern

If your reserves of cool, calm energy become "hot." In the view of natural medicine, overheated blood becomes wild and "boils over," finding any outlet it

---

TREATMENT FOR WEAK PATTERN OF HEAVY PERIODS

Herbs

Note: See p.38 for doses and cautions for herbs.
● During your period take Shepherd's purse (*Capsella bursa-pastoris*), Cranesbill (*Geranium maculatum*), False unicorn root (*Chamaelirium luteum*), and Beth root (*Trillium pendulum*), as a combined prescription.
● At other times take the same prescription, and add Licorice *(Glycyrrhiza glabra)* and Gentian (*Gentiana lutea*).
  Shepherd's purse may help to stem bleeding, Cranesbill is a general astringent, and False unicorn root and Beth root are uterine tonics.
● Lady's mantle (*Alchemilla vulgaris*) may be used instead of Shepherd's purse.

Homeopathy

Note: See p.54 for doses and cautions for homeopathic remedies.
● If you find it difficult to show affection, and you feel a dragging sensation in the lower abdomen - Sepia.

● If you sense a lack of emotional support, and you are generally anxious, with nasal and vaginal discharges between your periods - Calc. carb.

Exercises

Note: See p.70 for details of exercise routines.
● Weak routine.
  In addition:
● Swimming frog. Lie on your back, hands in the "praying" position at your chest, knees bent, and soles together. Exhale and straighten your arms and legs in opposite directions, raising your feet off the floor. Stretch and point your toes forward, like a frog swimming powerfully across a pond. Inhale and return to the starting position. Continue these movements rhythmically for 2-3 minutes, until you feel your lower trunk has done some work, then lie back and relax.

Swimming frog

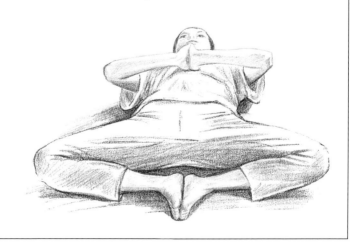

can, such as menstrual bleeding and possibly nosebleeds. A nosebleed can often be stemmed by applying a cold compress, but external cold applications are not usually effective for heavy menstrual bleeding (although some herbal applications are). Since you must not only take away excessive heat, but also supply positive, calm energy, external cold applications are ineffective.

Causes for this pattern are the factors which deplete cool energy. The problem often lies in trying to fit too many demands into an already crowded life. You may find yourself taking stimulants such as tea, coffee, and alcohol, to help you to keep going - but they do not increase underlying energy reserves. This pattern is also common at the menopause and in painful periods.

Symptoms Typically, the lack of cool energy pattern reveals itself as follows:
■ the blood is brilliant red,
■ bleeding is worse if you become excited or stimulated,
■ you may gain comfort from a hot water bottle on the lower abdomen,
■ the problem is generally worse when you become too hot, drink alcohol, or take stimulants,
■ your periods are regular, often coming early, and
■ your apparently energetic outlook relies on stimulants, and you become extremely tired as soon as you relax or unwind.

"Hot" pattern

In this pattern, heavy bleeding occurs because your body has accumulated too much heat. In a high fever, if blood and heat rush to the head, you get a throbbing headache. If the heat goes down it can have a similar effect on the uterus, and the blood flows out in quantity.

The multitude of factors leading to heat (see p.27) cause this pattern. On the physical level they include hot weather, especially if you have difficulty in perspiring; eating "hot" foods (see p.33); drinking alcohol; and long-term effects of an infectious disease, even from years previously. On the emotional level there are "hot" emotions such as anger, frustration, and sexual stimulation.

GENERAL ADVICE FOR HEAVY PERIODS

● If you have lost a large amount of blood, the homeopathic remedy China should help to restore your body's balance.
● Prepare a herbal skin application from Shepherd's purse (*Capsella bursa-pastoris*), Cranesbill (*Geranium maculatum*), and Tormentil (*Potentilla tormentilla*). Moisten the dried herbs into a poultice, or pour the tinctures onto a cotton pad. Then apply the poultice or pad to the area over the uterus, for 5-10 minutes, 3 times daily. Try this for a few days before the period and while it lasts.
● Above all, rest during your period. Take things easy, spend a quiet hour after your midday meal, and respect the demands of your body. Rest at the right time, and you will be twice as effective during the following month.
● It may take several cycles before your periods settle down, and up to a year if you previously had heavy periods for many years.

Symptoms The usual features of the hot pattern are as follows:

- bleeding is sudden and violent,
- the blood is often dark and clotted,
- you cannot reduce the blood flow either by lying down (which only makes you restless) or by placing a hot water bottle on the area,
- you have trouble keeping cool,
- your periods usually come several days early (your cycle is less than 28 days), and
- you have a dynamic, restless temperament, but you avoid stimulants, and may prefer vegetarian food. (Treatment for this pattern is given on p.118.)

"Blockage" pattern

In this pattern, your normal energy circulation becomes obstructed. The blockage is usually rather general (see p.25), and causes aches, pains, and other symptoms all over the body, which indicate energy is not moving freely. When energy becomes blocked in your uterus, menstrual bleeding then becomes painful and irregular.

On the physical level, this pattern is linked to excessive mental activity without balancing physical activity and exercise. Your emotional state is particularly important in this pattern. In particular,

---

TREATMENT FOR LACK OF COOL PATTERN OF HEAVY PERIODS

Herbs

Note: See p.38 for doses and cautions for herbs.
- Lady's slipper (*Cypripedium pubescens*), Yarrow (*Achillea millefolium*), and Motherwort (*Leonurus cardiaca*), as a combined prescription.

Lady's slipper reduces agitation, and Yarrow is a tonic and regulator that may also help to stop bleeding and reduce heat. Motherwort balances the prescription.

Other useful herbs are:
- Water lily (*Nymphaea alba*).
- Passion flower (*Passiflora incarnata*).
- Rue (*Ruta graveolens*).

Homeopathy

Note: See p.54 for doses and cautions for homeopathic remedies.

The following remedies may make you feel slightly depressed and prone to headaches at first, but this should soon give way to calm cheerfulness.
* Caution: Never use Phosphorus and Nit. ac. at the same time. They may interact to worsen the problem.
- If your eyes, ears, and other senses are extremely delicate, and you tend to be jumpy - Phosphorus.*
- If you tend to twitch on going to sleep, you have skin boils, and you talk compulsively - Lachesis.

- If you have sore sensations around your body, you had problems after childbirth, and you nurse grievances - Nit. ac.*
- If you are pale and weak, with a nervous disposition, and you blush easily - Ferr. met.
- If you have lost body fluids, the blood is very dark, you have developed long-standing conditions after childbirth, and you tend to "give" yourself to those around - China.

Exercises

Note: See p.70 for details of exercise routines.
- Easy routine.
- Waterball visualization (see p.126).

TREATMENT FOR HOT PATTERN OF HEAVY PERIODS

Herbs

Note: See p.38 for doses and cautions for herbs.
- Shepherd's purse (*Capsella bursa-pastoris*), Marigold petals (*Calendula officinalis*), Sage (*Salvia officinalis*), and Bearberry (*Arctostaphylos uva-ursi*). Shepherd's purse stems bleeding, and Marigold and Sage clear the heat. Bearberry cools the urinary tract, so that if the urine becomes acidic, there is less risk of inflammation and cystitis (see p.179).
- Lady's mantle (*Alchemilla vulgaris*) may be used instead of Shepherd's purse.

Homeopathy

Note: See p.54 for doses and cautions for homeopathic remedies.
- If you suffer thumping headaches, you feel physically and mentally confined, and your whole face is red - Belladonna.
- If the bleeding is painful and happens between periods, and parts of your face are red - Borax.

Exercises

Note: See p.70 for details of exercise routines.
- Strong routine, to dissipate heat.
- Brandysnap breathing (see p.118). Sit comfortably with your back straight. Open your mouth and curl your tongue into the tube-like brandysnap shape. Breathe long and deep through the brandysnap, making each breath in the same length as a breath out, by imagining a ticking clock, for 5-10 minutes.

if you habitually repress your feelings and have no outlet or expression for them, the resulting emotional blockage may lead to an energy blockage.

Symptoms of this pattern include:
- the menstrual bleeding is irregular, sometimes better and sometimes worse,
- the blood often has clots and varies in colour from dark to pale,
- it becomes worse if you sit still, and improves when you get moving,
- you may have pain,
- you can obtain relief from the warmth of a hot water bottle,
- your periods may be irregular, with vaginal discharge between, and
- the area under your right ribs (the site of your gall bladder) may be tender.

In the blockage pattern of heavy periods, there may be sensitivity or tenderness over the gall bladder area. This is linked to the "galling" repression of emotions and feelings.

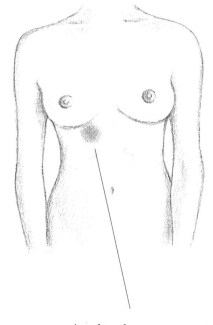

site of tenderness

TREATMENT FOR BLOCKAGE PATTERN OF HEAVY PERIODS

Diet

Avoid coffee and drink a soothing herbal tea, such as Chamomile (*Anthemis nobilis*).

Herbs

Note: See p.38 for doses and cautions for herbs.
- Shepherd's purse (*Capsella bursa-pastoris*), Motherwort (*Leonurus cardiaca*), Feverfew (*Chrysanthemum parthenium*), and Lobelia (*Lobelia inflata*).
- If you have difficulty digesting fats - add Fringe tree (*Chionanthus virginica*) and Balmony (*Celone glabra*).
   Shepherd's purse stops bleeding, Motherwort is a relaxant and energy regulator, Feverfew helps to move energy and bring down heat, and Lobelia is a general relaxant.

Homeopathy

Note: See p.54 for doses and cautions for homeopathic remedies.
- If you are very irritable and have cramping pains - Chamomilla.
- If the blood is dark and clotted or sticky - Crocus.
- If you have a red face, you tend to overwork in your chosen career, your periods are irregular with dark, clotted blood, and you suffer constipation, nausea, and irritation - Nux vomica.
- If you tend to burst into tears, and show a very warm, receptive personality - Pulsatilla.
- If you have lost body fluids, the blood is very dark, you have developed long-standing conditions after childbirth, and you tend to "give" yourself to those around - China.

Exercises

Note: See p.70 for details of exercise routines.
- Strong and Dynamic routines on alternate days.

In addition:
- Lizard. Practise the twisting movement gradually, reaching farther each time.
   Sit on the floor with legs apart. Lean your hands on the floor by one hip. Bend the knee on that side until the foot nears your groin. Lean more on your hands as you stretch the other leg straight out behind, twisting the foot sole-up. Each time you exhale, lean a little farther, stretching your flanks and inner legs. Continue for 60-90 seconds. Exhale as you untwist to the starting position. Repeat the whole exercise on the other side.

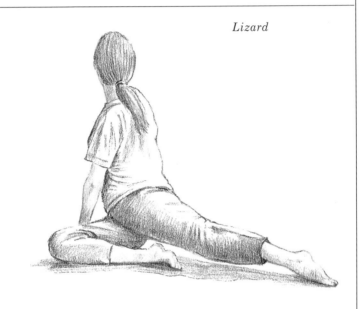

Lizard

IRREGULAR PERIODS

In an average cycle, periods come every 28 days or so, and each period is generally of the same length. (In some families, there is a tendency to a slightly longer or shorter cycle than the "standard" 28 days.) There are three common patterns of irregular periods which cause problems: those where the cycle is unpredictable, sometimes more than 28 days and sometimes less; periods that are always early; and those that are late .

Unpredictable periods

Some women have periods which are really irregular, being sometimes a few days early, and at other times a few days late. In extreme cases there may be intervals of only two weeks between periods, or as long as three months. This irregularity is especially common at the menopause (see p.168).

There are usually two main factors involved. One is the energy in the reproductive system (and often the whole of the pelvic region), which is weak - not weak enough to cause pathological problems, but more of a constitutional tendency. Just as some people have

CAUTIONS

Delayed or absent periods may be due to other conditions, including:
- coming off the contraceptive pill,
- extreme activity or exercise, as in athletes and ballet dancers,
- anorexia nervosa,
- imbalance of thyroid hormones, or
- polycystic disease of the ovaries.
Before you begin treatment, consider such causes. If in doubt, consult a physician of orthodox medicine.

strong muscles and others weak ones, so some people have more energy in the reproductive organs, and others possess relatively little energy there.

The other component involves strong feelings and emotions. A woman with this constitution is often sensitive and has mood swings. A disheartening event pulls her right down, while a more positive event brings on great thrills and excitement. These strong emotions interact with the energy in the reproductive system, causing hormonal levels to fluctuate. When she is excited or stimulated, the periods come early; if she is bored or depressed, they are late.

This problem tends to affect those whose work or activity is chiefly mental. The mental processes concentrate energy in the head, leaving reduced amounts in the lower part of the body. This leads to the characteristic feature of difficulty in interacting with the physical world. Natural remedies can help in the short term, but in the long term, compensating physical activity is needed to draw energy back down to the abdomen. Horse-riding, tennis, gardening, and similar sports and activities are particularly recommended.

Early periods

There are two common patterns here, and the causes and treatment are different. If you cannot decide which one applies to you, consult a practitioner.

"Full heat" pattern The early period is due to excess heat in the body, which makes the blood too "hot." It becomes overactive, like an imaginary boiling cauldron, and the extra pressure forces it out of its normal pathways.

TREATMENT FOR UNPREDICTABLE PERIODS

Diet

Try a diet with plenty of raw vegetables. Often, eating raw vegetables for two out of three meals each day brings a dramatic improvement. (However, take care not to become anaemic, see p.93.)

Herbs

Note: See p.38 for doses and cautions for herbs.
- Chaste tree (*Vitex agnus-castus*) is the herb of choice. Take it either as pills, or as 20 drops of tincture in water, 3 times daily.
- Other herbs which can help are Mugwort (*Artemisia vulgaris*), Motherwort (*Leonurus cardiaca*), or Rue (*Ruta graveolens*), taken singly or in combination.

Homeopathy

Note: See p.54 for doses and cautions for homeopathic remedies.
- If you tend to burst into tears, and dislike fatty foods - Pulsatilla.
- If you take more interest in mental rather than physical matters - Sulphur.
- If you tend to depression, grieving, and sadness, and to watery discharges and colds - Nat. mur.
- If you are tired from too much mental work - Actea.
- If you crave sweets, find sex painful, suffer from diarrhoea, and are generally fearful - Arg. nit.
- If you are often drowsy, and have pain at the base of your spine - Nux moschata.

Take homeopathic remedies 3 times daily at low (6X) potencies, or infrequently at high potencies (see p.56).

Mineral salts

- The mineral salt Selenium is sometimes helpful. (Mineral salts are similar to their corresponding homeopathic remedies, but are prepared differently. Ask at your local health store or pharmacy.)

There are many causes of this pattern. At the basic physical level it can be due to getting too hot, to a severe fever (some women get a period every time they have influenza), or to a family tendency to hot-pattern illnesses (see p.27).

Typical symptoms include:
- your period is up to seven days early, with heavy bleeding and clots,
- you may have bleeding between periods, when tired or overworked,
- a tendency to nosebleeds,
- a red face,
- you feel worse in very hot weather, and prefer cooling foods (see p.32), and
- you are generally restless, with difficulty in sleeping, and quick to anger. (Treatment is described on p.122.)

"Lack of cool" pattern This pattern is more common in the West than in the East, and is characteristic of nervous exhaustion. Again, the cause for the early bleeding is thought to be "hot blood," but in this case the blood has become heated by using all of the natural "coolness" in the body. It is analogous to a car that has lost all the cooling fluid from its radiator and cooling system, and thus soon overheats.

In contrast to the full heat pattern, where you may be able to trace the problem back to a clear cause, there may well be no obvious beginning to the lack of cool pattern. Your body's natural "coolness" may simply be used up over a long period of time. The commonest reason for this is fatigue from overstimulation. You may be stimulated from without, as when leading a very exciting life, or by some inner cause, when your willpower drives you on even after you are very tired. In both cases, your will forces your body beyond its normal strength and stamina.

Typical symptoms of the lack of cool pattern include:
■ you have red cheeks, but the rest of your face is pale,
■ your forehead is hot,
■ your skin is dry,

■ the periods are up to seven days early, and even earlier when you are tired,
■ the blood is bright red, and
■ bleeding may be heavy or light.

General advice The same advice applies to both patterns, although the lack of cool pattern is generally not so food-sensitive (see Treatment, p.124). The most effective action is to alter your lifestyle, so that you no longer need to rely on stimulants. A change which seems simple, but is often extremely difficult to carry out,

TREATMENT FOR FULL HEAT PATTERN OF EARLY PERIODS

This pattern can often be cured by change in lifestyle, without recourse to medicines. First, avoid all heating foods (see p.33), in particular red meat, alcohol, spicy foods, and stimulants as in coffee and tea. Take steps to disperse the heat by regular vigorous exercise and saunas.

Take herbal remedies for about 10 days before the expected date of the period, ideally from ovulation, if you know this date. Homeopathic remedies may be taken from the same time at the usual 6X potencies, or infrequently at higher potencies (see p.56).

Herbs

Note: See p.38 for doses and cautions for herbs.
● Marigold (*Calendula officinalis*), Sage (*Salvia*

officinalis), and Shepherd's purse (*Capsella bursa-pastoris*). Marigold clears heat from the body, Sage regulates its systems, and Shepherd's purse helps to control excessive bleeding.
● If you also feel weak, add Yarrow (*Achillea millefolium*) to the above prescription.
● During your period, make a compress of the following herbs, and apply it to your lower abdomen - Shepherd's purse, Marigold.

Homeopathy

Note: See p.54 for doses and cautions for homeopathic remedies.
● If you are stressed, irritable, and easily angered, with a red face, and possibly nausea and PMS (PMT) - Nux vomica.
● If you fear falling, your

periods are painful, and the symptoms are worse with wine or vinegar - Borax.
● If all of your senses are very delicate, you have heat throughout your body, and you tend to abdominal colic before your period, and pounding headaches - Belladonna.
● If you are irritable or jealous, with pain on ovulation, and urine retention with stinging sensations - Apis mel.
● If your menstrual flow is dark, with clots, and increases when you lie down - Cactus.

Exercises

Note: See p.70 for details of exercise routines.
● Strong routine, plus Bow (see p.112), Brandysnap breathing (see p.118), and Pelvic balancer (see p.107).

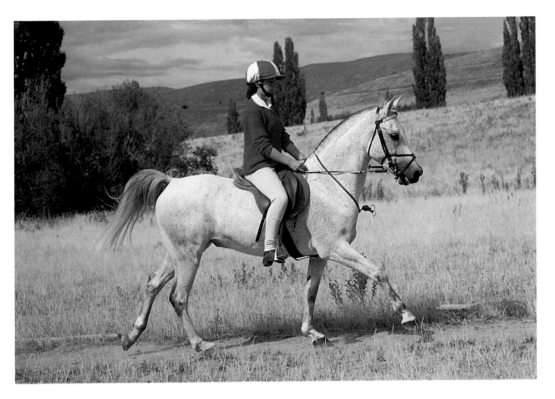

is to be less committed in your life, especially to others. Take more time off and spend it relaxing. And make some space for yourself, to build up calm and serenity in your life.

Late periods (and no periods)

Just as there are two main patterns for early periods, there are two common patterns for late periods.

If your periods are consistently late, or even absent, but you have no symptoms of either pattern - in fact, you might feel well most of the time - this indicates a problem at a higher level of existence (see p.15), which may not respond to natural medicines. In such cases, psychological and spiritual assistance may be more appropriate.

Factors which slow energy circulation can affect the periods. A common example is lack of physical exercise. Activities such as horse-riding improve posture (see p.85) and help to draw energy down to the lower abdomen.

"Blockage" pattern In this pattern of later periods, you are basically strong and healthy, but for some reason the periods do not come. The fundamental cause is blockage on the energy level; it may affect your overall energy circulation, or be a local blockage in the uterus itself.

On the physical level, any factor which slows energy circulation can affect the periods. Most common are overeating (especially rich foods), too many alcoholic drinks, and too little compensating physical exercise. Another common physical cause is recurrent constipation,

123

TREATMENT FOR LACK OF COOL PATTERN OF EARLY PERIODS

For general advice, see Treatment for the full heat pattern, p.122.

Herbs

Note: See p.38 for doses and cautions for herbs.
● Lady's slipper (*Cypripedium pubescens*), Yarrow (*Achillea millefolium*), and Beth root (*Trillium pendulum*). Lady's slipper calms and reduces tension, Yarrow is a tonic and reduces heat and sweating, and Beth root is a uterine tonic. Take this combination of herbs throughout the month.
● If your emotions are unstable, add Motherwort (*Leonurus cardiaca*) to the above prescription.

● The Chinese patent pills "8 Treasures" or "Women's precious" may help.

Homeopathy

Note: See p.54 for doses and cautions for homeopathic remedies.
* Caution: Never use Nit. ac. and Phosphorus at the same time. They may interact to worsen the problem.
● If you are very excited, and your period is long and heavy, with bright red blood - Phosphorus.*
● If you have sensations of soreness, and problems began after childbirth or miscarriage - Nit. ac.*
● If you are irritable and nervous - Bryonia.
● If your period is dark,

with dark clots, and you generally feel weak and shaky - China.
● If your period is long and heavy, and you are excitable and blush easily - Ferr. met.
  Take the homeopathic remedies 3 times daily at normal potencies, or infrequently at high potencies (see p.56).

Exercises

Note: See p.70 for details of exercise routines.
● Waterball visualization routine (see p.126).
● In addition, practise long, deep breathing. Aim to restore rhythm in yourself by equalizing inhalations and exhalations, done to the imaginary tick of a clock or metronome.

which reduces energy circulation in the whole of the lower abdomen, thereby influencing the periods. Sometimes the period is delayed by "cold" entering the body, as from cold weather or catching a chill. Just as heat makes periods come early, cold tends to "freeze" the inside of the body and delay the normal flow.

One effect of lovemaking is to slow the energy circulation in the uterus (see p.127). This is a normal reaction; strong energy flow would transport a fertilized egg out of the uterus before it had time to implant. It is quite common for women to have a delayed period after particularly passionate union.

On the emotional plane, frustration and anger are particularly likely to stagnate energy. More generally, any emotion which does not find an outlet or expression can cause stagnation. So if you feel frustrated or irritated, but have no way of giving vent to these feelings, they can stay bottled up inside - as can the period. The common symptoms are:
■ the period can be days or weeks late,
■ you have sensations of fullness, often a bloated lower abdomen and swollen, tender breasts, as though a period is about to start,
■ you feel irritable and fed up before the period begins, and

■ you are relieved when the period finally begins, even though it may be painful during the first day or two.

"Weak" pattern In this pattern, the periods are late because your body is weak, and possibly anaemic; it retains body fluids and blood for as long as possible, since their loss causes further depletion.

This common pattern is often due to long periods of exhaustion, with too much to do and not enough rest; you have no spare energy to make blood. It is closely linked to insufficient blood and anaemia, and the emotional features of this pattern are similar to those described on p.96. You may feel that all your energy is draining away, like water disappearing into sand, with no way to replenish it. You may have become so dragged down by material cares, that your "bubbling spring" of spiritual energy has dried up, and there is nothing to lift your soul to a higher plane. The symptoms clarify the picture:

■ you are tired most of the time,
■ your pale face has dark-ringed eyes,
■ the periods are many weeks late, and
■ when they eventually come, they increase your tiredness and fatigue.

TREATMENT FOR BLOCKAGE PATTERN OF LATE PERIODS

This pattern usually responds well to natural medicine. Take herbal remedies for about 10 days before the expected date of your period, ideally from ovulation, if you know its date. Homeopathic remedies may be taken in the usual low potencies this way, or infrequently at high potencies (see p.56).

Herbs

Note: See p.38 for doses and cautions for herbs.
● Blue cohosh (*Caulophyllum thalactroides*) or Black cohosh (*Cimicifuga racemosa*). Caution: Do not take either of these herbs if you are planning pregnancy, since they may affect egg implantation in the uterus.

● Cramp bark (*Viburnum opulus*) and Valerian (*Valeriana officinalis*). Cramp bark moves the energy in the uterus and reduces spasms; Valerian is an energy-mover.
● If you are agitated and have PMS (PMT), add Catmint (*Nepeta cataria*) to the above prescription.
● Mild cases respond well to Chamomile (*Anthemis nobilis*), 1 cup of tea daily.

Homeopathy

Note: See p.54 for doses and cautions for homeopathic remedies.
● If you suffer itching, skin irritation, and discharges, you are chilly and overweight, and you have a timid, uncertain nature - Graphites.

● If you often feel angry, irritable, and restless - Chamomilla.
● If you are prone to tears, your legs feel heavy, and there is a creamy vaginal discharge - Pulsatilla.
● If you tend to hold onto your feelings, and you have a swollen lower abdomen, often with constipation and flatulence - Lycopodium.
● If your periods seem to be delayed by fright or chills - Aconite.
● If the flow is only during the daytime - Causticum.

Exercises

Note: See p.70 for details of exercise routines.
● Strong or Dynamic routine - but you should do this daily.

TREATMENT FOR WEAK PATTERN OF LATE PERIODS

Treatment will succeed only if you can identify and rectify the causes of your exhaustion and energy depletion. However, natural remedies bring a sense of vigour that helps to reveal where your energy is being lost. Do not take remedies during your period, unless advised otherwise.

Herbs

Note: See p.38 for doses and cautions for herbs.
• False unicorn root (*Chamaelirium luteum*), Beth root (*Trillium pendulum*), Yarrow (*Achillea millefolium*), and Motherwort *(Leonurus cardiaca).* The first two are tonics for the uterus, Yarrow is a general tonic, and Motherwort regulates the periods. These remedies may be taken at all times of the month.

Homeopathy

Note: See p.54 for doses and cautions for homeopathic remedies.
• If you are very exhausted, experience "bearing-down" sensations, and are unable to show feelings - Sepia.
• If your glands are swollen, and you feel bruised but with no physical cause - Conium.

• If your willpower drives your body too hard - Silica.
• If you are preoccupied by mental activity and ideas, and you have skin eruptions and itching - Sulphur.
• If you are pale and lethargic, with a weak digestion, and fear the dark - Carbo veg. or Alumina.
   Take the remedies 3 times daily at the normal 6X potencies, or infrequently at high potencies (see p.56).

Exercises

Note: See p.70 for details of exercise routines.
• Weak or Easy routine. In addition:
• Waterball visualization. Lie relaxed on your back, and rest your awareness inside your abdomen, halfway between navel and spine. Without abruptness, visualize a ball of lukewarm water in this position; dwell on it for some seconds. Then imagine the ball separating into two halves, that flow slowly into your hips, down the middle of your legs, to your feet. They then move back up to your lower back, up along your spine, outward through your shoulders, down your arms into your hands, and back up to your neck. Here they coalesce into one, gently move up into the top of your

head, returning through your forehead, face, and throat, to the start. Finally, the ball expands as it fills your body with soft, luke-warm water. You may wish to visualize a ball of warm, glowing light rather than water. Time: 3-5 minutes.

The imaginary journey for waterball visualization

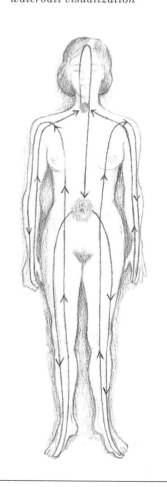

Conditions associated with Pregnancy

The huge amount of energy that love-making releases is the major factor, on the energy levels, that enables a new soul to enter the world. In the first weeks after conception, there is very little on the physical plane that could be called a new life - just a few undifferentiated cells, although they have great potential. Nevertheless many women are conscious of having conceived the moment the new soul is created.

Conception to three months When you become pregnant, the developing embryo combines with changes in your body to alter the circulation of energy in your uterus (womb). In later weeks, the foetus will take almost all of the energy flowing into your uterus, and also many nutrients from your blood, both being essential for its growth. But at this early stage, it is too small in its physical body, and also in its "energy body," to absorb all the nutrients and energy flowing into your uterus. So, to prevent strong uterine energy discharging the tiny embryo at the next period, the energy in your uterus stagnates or is redirected upward. If your overall energy is not circulating well, this can have side-effects as energy pours up to your digestive organs. You may even experience signs of a continuing menstrual cycle, even to the extent of a slight show of blood.

This energy pattern, with stagnation in the uterus or redirection away from it, continues for about the first three months. After this, the foetus is large enough to absorb significant amounts of nutrients and energy. Thus your energy pattern changes after the first third of pregnancy, as energy again begins to flow strongly into your uterus. This is why women with a weak energy pattern may miscarry at this time (see p.131). As the fast-growing foetus takes all the available energy from your reproductive system, little is left to initiate cyclical changes, and so remaining traces of periods disappear after three months.

The developing embryo's major organs and systems form during the first three months, and it is very sensitive to the adverse effects of drugs, and also to the beneficial effects of a happy environment. You may be instinctively aware of this as, immediately after conception, you become extra-sensitive to negative factors such as tobacco smoke, alcohol, and poorly-prepared food.

After three months As the foetus continues to grow, your own energy becomes re-directed back to the uterus. This can be your most exhausting time, as the new baby helps itself to all that it needs. If you are in good health, you may not feel especially tired, but any problems with energy deficiency or anaemia may become more pronounced as your pregnancy proceeds.

Self-care in pregnancy

Ancient Chinese authorities advocated that a woman be very calm and quiet during pregnancy. She should surround herself with beautiful sights and sounds, letting her mind rest on uplifting thoughts. Pleasant though this sounds, it is hardly practical for most women in today's culture. So what is really important? What should you do and avoid?

With a knowledge of energy flows in pregnancy, you can identify the two most important precautions: get enough rest, and lead a calm life. Plenty of rest is the single most important piece of advice for

FOODS TO AVOID DURING PREGNANCY

● The Chinese consider that oranges contain a "poison" which leads to hyperactivity, a finding supported in our own children's clinics. Do not eat more than one orange, or its equivalent in juice, per week.
● Some seafoods, such as shrimps, crabs, and shellfish, may increase "poisons" that accumulate in pregnancy, and make a new baby prone to rashes and allergies.
● Avoid any food to which you have an allergy. Otherwise your baby may develop similar allergic tendencies.
● Highly seasoned or spiced foods, such as game, chilli, or curry, may strain the livers of mother and baby.
● Many of the herbs and spices used in curry, especially Saffron, have a strong effect on the uterus.
● Alcohol's detrimental effects on the unborn child are well known.

any pregnant woman. This means, quite simply, stopping when you feel tired. Many people are brought up to believe that they should continue being active for as long as possible, almost until exhaustion sets in. This attitude does not apply during pregnancy. It is a question of respect for the developing new life, which needs your energy.

The second piece of advice is to avoid too much stimulation. During the latter half of pregnancy, the baby's nervous system is maturing. If you stay calm and serene at this time, then when the baby is born, he or she should be calm, too. Conversely, if you become nervous or excited too often, your new baby may show the same tendencies. This is not an absolute rule, since each pregnancy is different. But our experience in children's health clinics shows that many babies are affected by the mother's emotional state during pregnancy.

Diet in pregnancy

During pregnancy, a woman's instincts are heightened. You will probably know exactly which foods you need. Some aspects of diet, however, can bypass the natural instincts.

Eat organically grown foods, if possible. The extra expense is worth it, especially during the first three months, when the developing embryo is very sensitive to traces of pesticides and other chemicals sometimes found in non-organic foods. Moreover, its new body requires relatively large quantities of trace minerals. Foods grown in impoverished soil may lack these minerals.

If organic foods are not available, consider taking vitamin and mineral supplements. Consult a practitioner of natural medicine or a diet expert for advice. Always check the package to ensure that the supplements you buy are safe for use during pregnancy.

Eat plenty of foods with available iron. This is important during the later stages of pregnancy, but the time to prepare is during the first half, when your body is building up reserves of iron, vitamin B12, folic acid, and other substances (see Anaemia, p.93).

For many women, pregnancy brings increased awareness of emotions and feelings, and greater confidence in their bodies' abilities to nurture a new life.

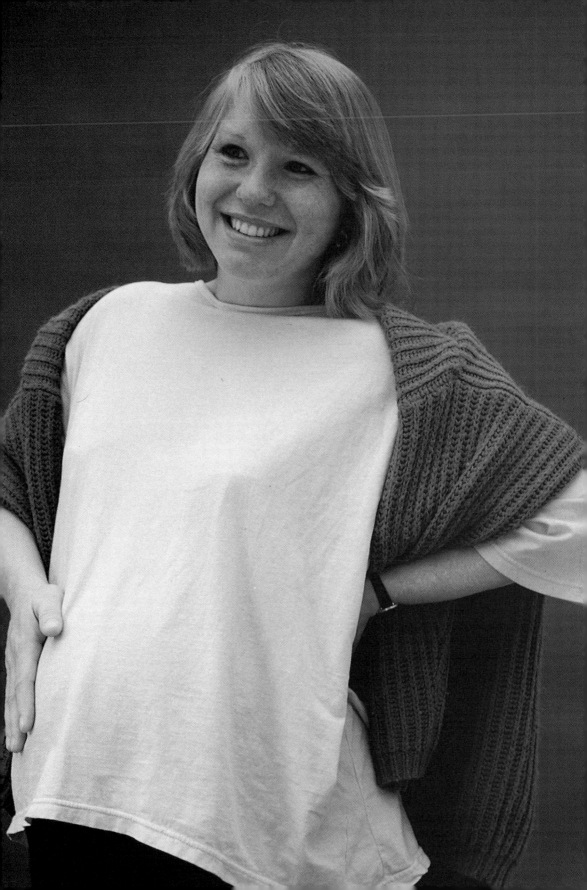

INFERTILITY (DIFFICULTY IN CONCEIVING)

While many women spend time and effort avoiding conception, others would like to have a baby but have difficulty conceiving. This problem is sometimes called "infertility." Better terms would be "subfertility" or "inability to conceive," since the condition is often treatable. Sometimes a physical problem is the cause, such as a malformed uterus, infection-scarred fallopian tubes, or a cyst. Other cases are due to functional or energy factors, and these can often be helped by natural medicines.

Physical causes

On the physical level, inability to conceive is sometimes the result of abnormal development or disease in the reproductive system, either of the woman or her partner. Consider this possibility first, by consulting a physician or gynaecologist. Irregular or absent periods may make it difficult to conceive (see p.120).

Functional or energy causes

If you experience normal periods, and according to orthodox medical criteria you are ovulating normally and have no other obvious bars to fertility, then consider functional or energy causes. Three possibilities are discussed here.

"Weak energy" pattern The main problem is lack of energy in the reproductive system. You may have enough energy to function adequately according to orthodox medical tests, but not enough vitality in the uterus to quicken a new life. This may be due to an overall lack of energy, when you often feel tired, or to a specific lack of energy in the reproductive system or lower abdomen.

> ## IT TAKES TWO
>
> Conception requires a healthy sperm to fertilize the egg. It may be that your partner has a low sperm count, or too many abnormal sperm. Or both of you could have lower-than-average fertility, and the combination is causing the difficulty. Always consider infertility as a couple, and investigate the condition together.

Underlying this pattern are the many factors that can lead to exhaustion and depletion - overwork, late nights, a previous difficult childbirth, termination of pregnancy, injury, and so on. One common cause is having to stand for lengthy intervals during the day.

Typical symptoms include:
■ you probably feel tired most of the time, but especially around 4 or 5 o'clock in the afternoon,
■ your back feels weak and sore,
■ you feel "empty" after a period,
■ your vaginal and anal muscles are sometimes weak, causing slight incontinence or prolapse (see p.153),
■ a watery vaginal discharge,
■ dull and dark-ringed eyes, and
■ irregular sleep.

"Excess mucus" pattern There is too much mucus (phlegm) in the whole body, or in the reproductive system in particular. Some mucus formation is essential for health. Its gentle flow toward the exterior is one way of cleansing and eliminating unwanted substances. However, in some cases the mucous membranes of the body produce too much mucus - as when your nose seems to drip continually. In

the reproductive system this may block the fallopian tubes, so that the egg cannot pass from the ovary to the uterus, or it may create a uterine lining which is too thick and hostile for the fertilized egg to become embedded.

Possible causes of this general illness pattern are discussed on p.31 and p.103. Symptoms of mucus overproduction are:

- your skin and hair are greasy,
- you tend to become overweight,
- there is a creamy vaginal discharge,
- you have a postnasal drip, or mucus (phlegm) on your chest, and
- you experience pain at ovulation time, usually an ache or pain in the ovaries .

"Poor energy circulation" pattern Your energy does not circulate well, leading to irregular flow and stagnant areas. In the reproductive system this affects mainly the ovaries and fallopian tubes. (The IUCD may disturb energy pathways in this way, see p.182.)

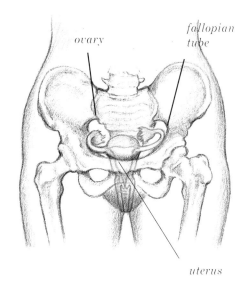

In the excess mucus pattern of fertility problems, there may be a characteristic ache in the ovaries around the time of ovulation. This is called "ovulation pain." The ovaries nestle in the curves of the hip bone, just above the level of the uterus.

MISCARRIAGE

Miscarrying during the first three months of pregnancy is very common. In many cases, the signs of pregnancy have not become established, and the miscarriage is not even recognized.

If this happens only once or twice, to your knowledge, it can be considered normal. Early miscarriage (also called spontaneous abortion) may be the body's way of getting rid of an abnormally developing embryo, or it happens because the uterine lining is not prepared to nurture the egg.

However, if you habitually miscarry during the first three months, or are in danger of miscarrying later in pregnancy, the cause may be an energy imbalance. The signs usually resemble the "weak energy" pattern of infertility, and precautions and treatment are the same. In particular:

- Rest is vital. Spend a quiet hour after your midday meal, lying back with your feet up.
- Do not take strenuous physical exercise, especially any activity that may strain your lower back.
- Avoid long periods of standing.
- If you have not already done so, cut out coffee, tobacco, and alcohol.

Poor energy in the ovaries disturbs their hormone secretions, which in turn leads to irregular periods - often without the release of an egg. The fallopian tube's normal wave-like muscular action, which helps to transport the egg, is also interrupted by low energy, and the egg is not carried to the uterus.

Among the causes of poor energy flow are suppressed emotions of anger, frustration, and bitterness. There are also the many tension-inducing factors of modern life - work deadlines, crowded streets, traffic stress, demands by partners, children and colleagues - without the balancing effect of calm, rhythmical, physical activity.

Typical symptoms of this pattern are:
■ your periods may be irregular and painful,
■ you feel frustrated and irritable, especially before periods, but better afterward, and
■ you usually feel better after some vigorous exercise.

Emotional and spiritual factors

Some women have no apparent physical problem, nor any significant energy imbalance, yet they still cannot conceive - even after orthodox and natural treatments. The cause may then be on a higher level, with something less tangible blocking the free flow of nutrients and energy. Consider the following paragraphs to see if you recognize your own situation, which can then guide you toward effective help.

Creative work Conceiving a new baby is the most creative activity imaginable. But creative energy (see p.18) is limited, and to a certain extent, you can direct it

and use it in other activities. If you have great demands in your job, or family situation, or social life, which require you to concentrate all of your creative energies every day, there may not be enough energy left to nourish a new life.

Blockage of creative energy Some couples who wish to conceive, but who have been unsuccessful, find that they are trying harder and harder. You may make careful notes to pinpoint your time of ovulation, and have special arrangements for lovemaking during your most fertile period. But such an intense effort and concentration may actually create stress and tension, that blocks or obstructs energy in the uterus, and so contributes to the difficulty in conceiving. It is rather like being so anxious about making a public speech, that you stiffen up and forget your words!

The key to overcoming the problem is learning to relax. Try to enjoy the phase you are in now, and relish life as it is. Focus on what you have got, rather than feeling empty about what you lack. This should help you to release tension, and allow warmth and relaxation to spread through your body.

Other emotional problems Just as you can become tense and so disturb your energy flow by trying too hard for a baby, so other tensions can interfere with conception. For example, deeply buried guilt and anxiety can affect the circulation of energy in your reproductive system. A discussion of these problems is beyond the scope of this book, but if natural medicines do not help, consider other methods. Psychoanalysis or counselling can help you come to terms with suppressed or hidden feelings.

TREATMENTS FOR INFERTILITY

It is an awesome thought that a herbal or homeopathic remedy, combined with exercises, and changes in lifestyle and attitude, could open the way for bringing a new life into the world. Nevertheless, simple actions based on identifying the correct pattern of the problem are often effective.

General advice

Try the remedies advised here for at least 3 months, even a year. During this time, take steps to avoid becoming pregnant, since pregnancy while taking treatment may result in a miscarriage. However, avoid the contraceptive pill, IUCD, or spermicidal cream if possible, and use another method.

Herbs

Note: See p.38 for doses and cautions for herbs.
● Chaste tree (*Vitex agnuscastus*) may be added to all the prescriptions below (see p.53).
● For the weak pattern - Beth root (*Trillium pendulum*), False unicorn root (*Chamaelirium luteum*), Yarrow (*Achillea millefolium*), and Licorice (*Glycyrrhiza glabra*). Beth root and False unicorn root strengthen the pelvic area

and reproductive system, Yarrow is a general tonic for the body and helps to regulate periods, while Licorice is an energy-mover.
● For the mucus pattern - Motherwort (*Leonurus cardiaca*), Golden seal (*Hydrastis canadensis*), Berberis (*Berberis vulgaris*), and Balmony (*Celone glabra*). Golden seal and Berberis clear mucus from the reproductive system, and Balmony stimulates the digestion and helps to clear the uterus of stagnant energy. Motherwort opens the way for the other herbs to work in this area.
● If you have indigestion, add Fringe tree (*Chionanthus virginica*) and Black root (*Leptandra virginica*).
● For the blockage pattern - Blue cohosh (*Caulophyllum thalactroides*), Motherwort (*Leonurus cardiaca*), and Catmint (*Nepeta cataria*). Blue cohosh moves energy in the reproductive system, Motherwort helps regulate the periods, and Catmint gently warms the reproductive organs.

Homeopathy

Note: See p.54 for doses and cautions for homeopathic remedies.
   Constitutional treatment under the guidance of a

homeopath is especially recommended for fertility problems (see p.56).
   For the weak energy pattern:
● If you have a dragging sensation in the uterus area, feel unable to show emotions, and experience a vaginal discharge before your period - Sepia.
● If you lack support from those around, have problems digesting milk, and dislike cold and wet weather - Calc. carb.
● If you have negative attitudes, watery discharges, fluid retention, and dislike lovemaking - Nat. mur.
● If you have fears of falling, a low sex drive, and a heavy vaginal discharge - Borax. In addition to constitutional doses, take 2 tablets of 3X potency before lovemaking.
   For the excess mucus pattern:
● If you suffer swollen mucous membranes, bad-smelling yellow discharges, a pale face that tends to develop spots, and frequent mental exhaustion - Mercurius.
● If you feel chilly yet lazy, frequently catch skin infections, and have white discharges - Graphites.
● If you feel emotionally

Continued on next page

Continued from previous page

injured, your face is hot, and the discharges are yellow and burning - Kreasotum.

For the poor energy circulation pattern or energy blockage:
● If you are generous, but impatient and prone to outbursts of rage - Chamomilla.
● If you feel uneasy with your femininity, and suffer muscle cramps - Viburnum.
● If you experience neuralgic pains - Cimicifuga.
● If you are very disappointed after lovemaking - Ignatia.
● If you have a strong sex drive, yet feel tired and sensitive, with a tendency to headaches - Lil. tig.

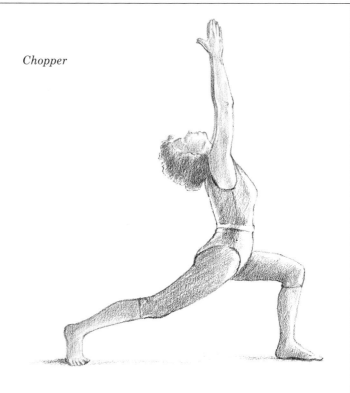

Chopper

Exercises

Note: See p.70 for details of exercise routines.

For the weak energy pattern:
● Emphasize exercises that improve kidney function, such as Plough (see p.77), Back stretch (see p.76), and Pelvic energizer (see p.104). In addition:
● Cobbler. This posture is named after the traditional Indian cobbler who held his work between his feet. Sit on the floor, knees bent outward, soles together. As you exhale, pull firmly on your feet with your hands, digging your elbows into your calves. With each further exhalation, pull slightly more. Feel your inner thighs and hips open, and a therapeutic stretch at the base of your back. Continue for 1-2 minutes, exhale slowly, and relax.
● Neckstand (see p.77) helps to redirect energy around the body, but do not do this during your period.

For the excess mucus and poor energy circulation patterns:
● Dynamic routine.
● In addition, Chopper. Stand with your feet fairly wide apart, and stretch your arms above your head, palms together. Turn your left foot outward at a right angle, and your right foot inward at 45º. Exhale as you twist your trunk to face left. Turn your right foot farther, raising your heel off the floor. Exhaling again, bend your left leg until its thigh is parallel to the floor. Drop your head back to gaze at your thumbs. Hold for 30-40 seconds. Exhale slowly as you resume the starting position, relax, and repeat on the other side. Feel the stretch along the front of your legs, and a twist at your flanks and back.

AFTER A TERMINATION

There may come a time when you find yourself unexpectedly pregnant, but because of your health and situation, you do not feel able to bring a child into the world. It is an extremely difficult decision to have a termination of pregnancy (TOP, also called a planned abortion, or simply "abortion"). There are

Talking to a good friend can help you to recognize, and come to terms with, your innermost feelings concerning a termination.

many arguments and views about the rights and wrongs of termination on health, moral, legal, and religious grounds. Most women are aware that they are preventing a newly-formed being from living a life; and the decision may appear to be based on selfish motives. There is a period of considerable inner turmoil during which the pros and cons are weighed carefully. However, there are usually strong reasons for a termination, including risks to health,

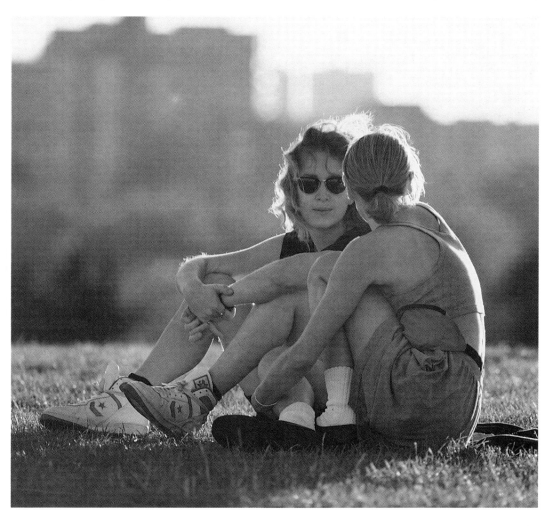

TREATING THE AFTER-EFFECTS OF TERMINATION

The first step in treatment must be spiritual. If your conscience is troubled, attend to this before carrying out work at lower levels. Persistent unease on the spiritual level can be helped by an experienced practitioner of natural medicine, a healer, or a group of people (religious or otherwise) who are working toward spreading love and healing in the world. Once you have sought spiritual guidance, other symptoms often become more amenable to treatment.

Many of the common physical effects are covered elsewhere in this book. For example, post-termination depression has certain parallels to postnatal depression (see p.158), and period problems are dealt with on pp.103-126. The natural remedies advised have their effects on the emotional level, too.

Deeper problems on the emotional level can be assisted by counselling, and various techniques of psychoanalysis, psycho-therapy, and psychiatric therapy. In many regions, there are self-help groups for those who suffer from emotional problems after a termination or other traumatic event.

Exercises

Note: See p.70 for details of exercise routines.

Our bodily functions rely on breathing, and nowhere is this more apt than when confronting grief. Thus, try the following:

- Regularly do long, deep breathing, equalizing the inhalations and exhalations, to bring calm and restore serenity. See the first exercise in the Dynamic routine, p.80.
- Sometimes you may find stronger breathing techniques helpful, for example, Bellows (see p.105) and Spike (see p.81).

Warning

Termination has been procured by taking large doses of certain herbs. However, this can have disastrous consequences, and should not be attempted. In most areas it is also unlawful.

difficult financial position, and the lack of a stable home - all of which may make it impossible for you to give a baby the love that it needs.

In most cases, the termination is carried out under anaesthetic, and so is painless at the time. Nevertheless, it is a traumatic intrusion of the body that has its effects on various levels. Physically, the abrupt ending of pregnancy greatly disturbs the hormonal system - not just the female hormones, but others. The resulting imbalance can make you feel exceedingly unwell. There may also be a risk of uterine or fallopian infection, and unforeseen effects on future fertility.

Emotionally, termination brings a complicated array of feelings. There may be relief at being liberated from health worries, to remorse at the loss of a life, to guilt at apparently "selfish" motives, and anger at acquiescing to the violation. It is hardly surprising that you may feel very upset for months, sometimes years, after. There may also be effects on the spiritual level. It can happen that a woman is aware of the spirit of the unborn child, years later. She may feel powerless to overcome these feelings, even though she is certain that her decision was right, and she may require appropriate counselling.

NAUSEA AND SICKNESS IN PREGNANCY

Nausea (feeling sick) and actual vomiting (being sick) are so common in early pregnancy, that many women view them as the first sure signs that they have conceived. The nausea often starts soon after the first missed period, and is frequently more severe in the morning - hence the name "morning sickness." Usually the sickness disappears after about three months. A few women are severely affected and their symptoms may last throughout the day, and even throughout pregnancy.

Severe nausea or vomiting can cause anxiety, since you may feel that the state of your body will affect your unborn baby. Surprisingly, adverse effects on the baby are exceedingly rare.

Causes

From the viewpoint of natural medicine, causes of nausea and vomiting are attributed to changes that occur when you become pregnant. First, the energy circulation in the uterus slows down (see p.127). Later in pregnancy, all the available energy and nourishment will be absorbed by the fast-growing foetus; but in the early stages uterine energy stagnates, to prevent the tiny embryo from being expelled at the time when the next period would be due. The normal downflow of energy that occurs during a period is redirected upward, to the digestive system.

What happens next depends on your state of energy circulation. If it is good, you should feel very well, because you can use the extra energy that would otherwise be lost in the period. If your overall energy circulation is poor, the digestive system slows down, leading to nausea in mild cases and vomiting in

more severe ones. Characteristically the symptoms are worse in the morning, when your energy flow is most sluggish. They tend to ease off after three months, as the growing baby absorbs significant amounts of energy and nutrients.

Emotional factors

Very strong emotions are released when you realize you have conceived. You may feel natural pride at the thought of creating a baby, and excitement at the prospect of changes ahead. But equally common and natural are a vague anger with the world in general or with your partner, for allowing it to happen, as well as fear of the unknown, worry at the reactions of your friends and relatives, and even despair at what the future might hold, and the thought of the effort involved in bringing up a child.

The interplay between such conflicting emotions produces a dislocation in the senses, which gives rise to nausea. You could compare it to a wild fairground ride, which arouses strong emotions and unsettles the senses in the same way, and produces the same effects.

Patterns of sickness

Morning sickness usually manifests itself in one of these three ways, depending on the cause of the stagnation in the digestive system.

"Weak stomach" pattern Typical symptoms of this pattern are:
■ your face is pale,
■ you have a poor appetite,
■ you are tired, and tend to anaemia,
■ you vomit mainly undigested food, and
■ you are generally anxious and fearful.

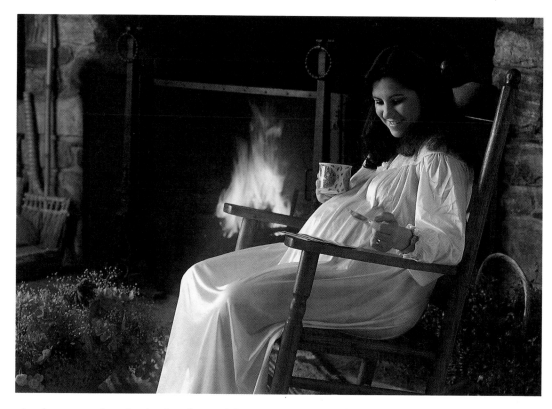

A calm approach and episodes of peaceful reflection help you to build good energy flow, thereby counteracting feelings of nausea due to energy stagnation in pregnancy.

"Blockage" pattern The typical symptoms of this pattern include:
- before pregnancy you had PMS (PMT), and liked coffee and alcohol,
- your face is yellowish,
- you have a tendency to headaches,
- you vomit yellow or green fluid after the food has come up, and
- you are easily angered or frustrated.

"Excess mucus" pattern The characteristic symptoms of this pattern are:
- you feel lethargic and "heavy,"
- you may be overweight,
- your skin is greasy, and your hair needs frequent washing,
- you vomit much watery fluid, and
- you have other signs of excess mucus, such as a runny nose.

General advice

The symptoms arise from poor energy circulation, so they are relieved when the energy flow revives. These pointers should help to restore good energy flow.
- A contributory factor to morning sickness is low blood sugar. This can be helped by a high-energy meal the night before, which keeps your blood sugar raised until morning.
- Do not eat in the morning until your energy is moving. As soon as you get up,

138

carry out an exercise routine as recommended on pp.72-81, or take a short walk.
● Then sip a warm drink, either plain hot water, or a mild tea such as Fennel seed tea (*Foeniculum vulgare*) sweetened with honey. This is also a good time to take any natural remedies.
● Eat easily digested foods, with plenty of fresh vegetables and available iron

(see p.93). Eat a light meal an hour or so before any daytime activity, to maintain good blood sugar levels.
● A stuffy atmosphere encourages feelings of nausea. Sleep with windows open, and keep them open during the day.
● Sensations of fear which often accompany the sickness can be helped by the Bach remedy Mimulus (see p.186).

TREATMENT FOR NAUSEA AND SICKNESS IN PREGNANCY

During the first 3 months, the developing embryo is at its most susceptible to any disturbances in body chemistry. Many mothers feel this instinctively, and take great care with what they eat and drink. This care naturally applies to medicines and herbs. The selected remedies given below have been used for centuries by pregnant women. However, should you suffer adverse reactions, stop the treatment at once and see a practitioner.

Herbs

Note: See p.38 for doses and cautions for herbs. Consult a herbalist before self-treatment.
● General prescription - Gentian (*Gentiana lutea*), Berberis (*Berberis vulgaris*), and Wild yam (*Dioscorea villosa*). This combination of herbs aids all types of sickness in pregnancy.

● For the weak stomach pattern - add False unicorn root (*Chamaelirium luteum*) to the prescription, and add Ginger and Fennel seed to food. Drink Lime tea (*Tilia europaea*).
● For the blockage pattern - add Balmony (*Celone glabra*), Fringe tree (*Chionanthus virginica*), and Valerian (*Valeriana officinalis*) to the prescription. Drink Chamomile tea (*Anthemis nobilis*).
● For the excess mucus pattern - add Oregon grape (*Berberis aquifolium*) to the prescription. Avoid milk, cheese, and peanut butter.

Homeopathy

Note: See p.54 for doses and cautions for homeopathic remedies. Consult a homeopath before self-treatment.
  For the weak stomach pattern:
● If you have a dragging sensation in the abdomen,

you dislike the sight or smell of food, and you feel that you cannot express emotions - Sepia.
● If you experience burning sensations, and want to withdraw from your present circumstances - Causticum.
● If your nausea is worse at night, and you have sour-tasting saliva and acid regurgitation into the gullet - Carbo animalis.
  For the blockage pattern:
● If you are energetic, fresh-faced, and with a strong driving force, and you feel a bad taste in your mouth - Nux vomica.
● If you have much suppressed anger, and your glands are enlarged and breasts sore - Conium.
● If you desire sweet foods yet cannot digest them well - Sulphur.
● If you are warm-hearted yet easily angered, and suffer cramps - Chamomilla.
● If you tend to burst into

Continued on next page

Continued from previous page

tears, suffer from yellow discharges, vomit night and day, and dislike meat and greasy foods - Pulsatilla.

For the excess mucus pattern:

● If you are sluggish, with a swollen abdomen, weak stomach, and mucous discharges from all orifices - Hydrastis.

● If you feel dizzy, have headaches and depression, and even thinking of food causes nausea - Cocculus.

● If you vomit all the time, salivate profusely, but feel better after eating - Lobelia.

● If you have a tendency to yellow burning discharges, and you vomit frequently but this does not make you feel better - Kreasotum.

Exercises

Note: See p.70 for details of exercise routines.

For the weak stomach pattern:

● Gondola. Sit with your legs straight in front, fingers interlocked behind your head. Lean back as you exhale, as far as you can, while gradually raising your legs off the floor. The upper abdominal contraction massages the stomach.

For the blockage pattern:

● Strong or Dynamic routine. In addition:

● Twisted angle. Sit with your legs straight in front,

Wounded soldier (starting position)

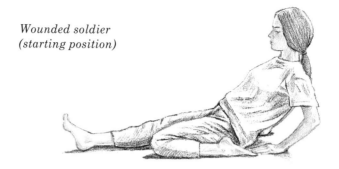

Wounded soldier (fully stretched position)

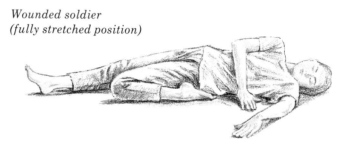

fairly wide apart. Exhale and lean your right shoulder toward the inside of your right knee. Let your left arm hang over your left ear and crown. If you can, pull on your right foot with both hands, to increase the twist. Remain for 30-60 seconds. Inhale deeply as you resume the starting position, and repeat on the other side.

For the excess mucus pattern:

● Dynamic or Strong routine, plus these two:

● Rib dig. Sit comfortably, and point your fingers slightly upward into your upper abdomen, just below your ribs, with palms up. Exhaling, lean forward until the backs of your hands

touch your thighs. Lean even farther, letting your thighs push your rigid hands into your stomach and liver area. Remain for 30-60 seconds, rest and relax, then repeat 2-3 times.

● Wounded soldier. If you are fairly supple, sit with one leg straight in front and the other tucked under your hip (first illustration). As you exhale, lean back onto the elbow of your bent-leg side, and reach for the floor with the opposite hand. Lean slightly more sideways with each breath, over 30-60 seconds (second illustration). Relax, then repeat on the other side.

OTHER PROBLEMS IN PREGNANCY

Many of the minor complaints of pregnancy can be helped by gentle, natural remedies. Some problems are caused by the way the baby is lying in the uterus, while others signify deeper imbalance. Pregnancy is not usually the best time to tackle deep-seated problems, but it is appropriate to settle the symptoms using such therapies as herbs, homeopathic treatments, and gentle exercises.

Many of the minor problems at this time stem from slight imbalances that predated conception; the extra stress of pregnancy causes them to develop into uncomfortable symptoms. For example, nosebleeds in pregnancy may be another manifestation of an imbalance that formerly led to heavy periods. The body is used to producing a lot of blood, and when you become pregnant, the normal outlet of the period ceases - consequently, you may have nosebleeds, possibly with raised blood pressure.

This section outlines the symptom patterns and remedies for common complaints during pregnancy. Further details of patterns and causes are given on the pages indicated. Refer to p.38 and p.54 for doses and cautions for herbs and homeopathic remedies respectively. See

CAUTION

Before you embark on self-treatment during pregnancy, consult a practitioner of orthodox medicine, who can exclude more serious conditions. Then take advice from the relevant herbalist or homeopath. Great care is needed when prescribing and estimating the doses of remedies for use during pregnancy.

p.70 for general information on the major exercise routines, and refer to the main Index on p.188 for page references to the individual exercises.

Palpitations and insomnia

Consult your family physician first, in case of an underlying heart condition.

For the lack of cool pattern (see p.98):
● Suitable herbs include Motherwort (*Leonurus cardiaca*), Beth root (*Trillium pendulum*), Yarrow (*Achillea millefolium*), and Passion flower (*Passiflora incarnata*).
● Homeopathic remedies include Phosphorus and Coffea.
● Rest is essential
● Exercises include Waterball visualization and the Weak or Easy routine.

If you have signs of the excess mucus pattern (see p.104):
● Herbs include Gentian (*Gentiana lutea*), Hawthorn (*Crataegus oxycantha*), and Oregon grape (*Berberis aquifolium*).
● Homeopathic remedies include Calc. carb. and Hydrastis.
● Avoid milk, cheese, and peanut butter in your diet.
● Exercises include Wounded soldier and Corner hang, and Chest, Middle, and Belly rocks from the Dynamic routine.

For the obstruction pattern (see p.108):
● Herbs include Gentian (*Gentiana lutea*), Fringe tree (*Chionanthus virginica*), Black root (*Leptandra virginica*), and Hawthorn (*Crataegus oxycantha*).
● Homeopathic remedies include Cimcifuga, Nux vomica, and Pulsatilla.
● Avoid rich, greasy foods and alcohol.
● Exercises include the Strong or Dynamic routine, plus Wall twist, Temple guardian, Sitting pretty, and Twisted angle.

High blood pressure

See a doctor, and consult a practitioner of natural medicine. Rest is essential. Yoga and/or meditation is usually very helpful (see p.82), as is a regular deep-breathing routine. In addition, do any of the exercises in this book which come naturally to you, preferably in a daily routine - but do not attempt any upside down positions.

Indigestion

See Nausea and sickness in pregnancy, p.137, for details of the symptom patterns and general advice, including exercises.

For the weak stomach pattern:
● Herbs include Gentian (*Gentiana lutea*), Berberis (*Berberis vulgaris*), and Wild yam (*Dioscorea villosa*).
● Homeopathic remedies include Calc. carb. and Causticum.
● Drink Fennel tea (*Foeniculum vulgare*), and cook food with Ginger (*Zingiber officinale*).

For the blockage pattern:
● Herbs include Fringe tree (*Chionanthus virginica*), Gentian (*Gentiana lutea*), Berberis (*Berberis vulgaris*), and Valerian (*Valeriana officinalis*).
● Homeopathic remedies include Pulsatilla and Nux vomica.
● Drink weak Chamomile tea (*Anthemis nobilis*).

Nosebleeds

See Period problems, pp.106-126, for details of the symptom patterns and general advice. In addition, arrange with your physician for an examination to make sure that you do not have raised blood pressure.

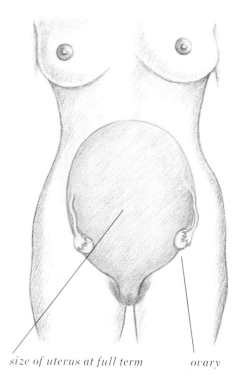

size of uterus at full term   *ovary*

During pregnancy, the uterus expands enormously to accommodate the growing foetus. As it compresses the other abdominal organs, this leads to digestive complaints.

For the obstruction pattern:
● Herbs include Shepherd's purse (*Capsella bursa-pastoris*), Feverfew (*Chrysanthemum parthenium*), Motherwort (*Leonurus cardiaca*), and Lobelia (*Lobelia inflata*).
● Homeopathic remedies include Nux vomica, Chamomilla, and Crocus sativa.

For the heat pattern:
● Herbs include Shepherd's purse (*Capsella bursa-pastoris*), Marigold petals (*Calendula officinalis*), Sage (*Salvia officinalis*), and Bearberry (*Arctostaphylos uva-ursi*).
● The main homeopathic remedy is Belladonna.

For the lack of cool pattern:
● Herbs include Lady's slipper (*Cypripedium pubescens*), Motherwort (*Leonurus cardiaca*), and Yarrow (*Achillea millefolium*).
● The main homeopathic remedy is Phosphorus.

Backache

See the descriptions of symptom patterns and the general advice given for Nausea and sickness in pregnancy, p.137. Your posture and the way you move and carry your baby are very important; obtain advice from a teacher of the Alexander technique (see p.85).

For the weak pattern:
● Herbs include Gentian (*Gentiana lutea*), Berberis (*Berberis vulgaris*), and Beth root (*Trillium pendulum*).
● Homeopathic remedies include Kali carb., Helonias, and Sepia.
● Take Fennel tea (*Foeniculum vulgare*).
● Exercises include Forward stretch, Moth, Cobbler, Swinging long stretch, and Leg stretch from the Weak routine.

For the obstruction pattern:
● Herbs include Fringe tree (*Chionanthus virginica*), Gentian (*Gentiana lutea*), Berberis (*Berberis vulgaris*), and Valerian (*Valeriana officinalis*).
● Homeopathic remedies include Bellis, Rhus tox, and Aesculus.
● Exercises include Lizard (see p. 119), Knee drop from the weak routine, and Leaning tower from the Easy routine.

Haemorrhoids (piles)

● Suitable herbs include Beth root (*Trillium pendulum*), Black root (*Leptandra virginica*), and Fringe tree (*Chionanthus virginica*).

● Homeopathic remedies include Lachesis, Sulphur, or Collinsonia when the piles protrude and you are very weak.

Urine retention

It is vital to consult a practitioner of orthodox medicine first, in case of a serious underlying cause.
● Herbs include Valerian (*Valeriana officinalis*), Beth root (*Trillium pendulum*), and Buchu (*Barosma betulina*).
● Homeopathic remedies include Eupatorium purp., Populus trem., and Sabal serrulata.
● Exercises include Great pull, Back stretch, and Forward stretch.

Constipation

Herbal remedies can help to relieve constipation during pregnancy, but take extra care, because of the slight risk of miscarriage. The herbs advised here move the energy in the lower part of the body, but first check with your physician in case of other problems, and then with a herbalist or homeopath before you start self-treatment. Never use high doses or a herbal purge.

For the weak pattern (see p.98):
● Suitable herbs include Gentian (*Gentiana lutea*) and Beth root (*Trillium pendulum*).
● Homeopathic remedies include Sepia, Causticum, and Collinsonia.

For the blockage pattern (see p.124):
● Herbs include Fringe tree (*Chionanthus virginica*), Balmony (*Celone glabra*), and Butternut (*Juglans cineria*). Feverfew (*Chrysanthemum parthenium*) may also be helpful.
● The main homeopathic remedy is Hydrastis.

143

For either pattern of constipation:
● Exercises include Hip swivel, Cobbler, Neckstand, and Plough.

Sore breasts

See also Breastfeeding problems, p.160. Consult a practitioner of orthodox medicine if the soreness persists for more than a few days, in case there is an abscess forming in the breast tissue.
● Herbs include Lobelia (*Lobelia inflata*), Wild yam (*Dioscorea villosa*), Fringe tree (*Chionanthus virginica*), and Poke root (*Phytolacca decandra*).
● There are several suitable homeopathic remedies, including Belladonna, Conium, Bryonia, and Pulsatilla.

SPECIAL EXERCISES FOR MINOR PROBLEMS IN PREGNANCY

Note: See p.70 for details of exercise routines.
● Corner hang. Stand with your feet fairly wide apart, in either a doorway or an open corner of the room. Extend your arms up at 45°. Supporting yourself with your hands on the door frame or walls, exhale and relax forward. Let your abdomen hang forward as much as possible. This will stretch you in a X shape from toes to fingers . With each exhalation, relax a little more forward. Finally, exhale deeply as you push on your hands and stand up again. Repeat 5-10 times over 2-3 minutes.
● Swinging long stretch. Lie on the floor on your back, with arms stretched out beyond your head, and legs straight. Exhaling, raise your hips off the floor, so that you are supported on your heels and shoulders. Push your heels forward, aiming your toes back. Exhaling, shift your hips sideways to the left. Inhale as you return them to the centre; exhaling, shift them sideways to the right. Repeat this 10-20 times.

Corner hang

Finally, exhale as you lower your hips and rest. This exercise will always feel awkward, but after you

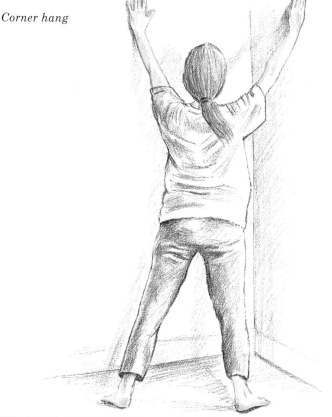

● Exercise positions include Laid back, Camel, Corner hang, and Twisted angle. Do not attempt exercises that increase the painful aching in the breasts.

Eczema

Relieve symptoms with herbal remedies, and consult a practitioner of natural or orthodox medicine concerning the underlying cause. In some cases, eczematous skin conditions are linked to increased allergic sensitivity during pregnancy.

● Herbs include Butternut (*Juglans cinerea*) at one quarter of the standard dose, or Burdock (*Arctium lappa*).

● Avoid cheese, milk, peanuts, oranges, coffee, red meat, and spicy foods.

---

should feel relief around your hips and lower back.

● Hip swivel. Stand with your feet shoulder-width apart, hands on hips. Rotate your hips in tiny circles. Gradually increase the diameter of the circles until your hips are moving outward in a large circle. Gradually diminish the circle's diameter again and come to an imperceptible halt. Then repeat all this, circling in the opposite direction. Let your awareness dwell on the delicate feelings in your lower back and hips.

● Laid back. Sit on the floor, either on your heels or with your buttocks between your heels. Exhaling, begin to lean back, supporting yourself behind with your hands. When you start to feel a strong stretch in your thighs, and perhaps in your belly, stay at that position for a few seconds. You may be able to lean back through several phases of this exercise: elbows on the

Laid back

ground; head dropping backward; crown on the floor, looking back; back on the ground, with arms stretched beyond your head. Throughout, keep your knees as close together as possible.

Stay in your preferred phase of this posture for anything from 30 seconds to 5 minutes. This exercise stretches your stomach channel from your toes, up along the front of your legs, abdomen, and breasts, to your throat.

● Slip-up. Lie on your back with your buttocks against a wall, supported on a cushion. Lean your legs on the wall and open them, exhaling, as wide as you can. Relax, letting the weight of your legs create a stretch along the insides of your thighs. Remain for 30-60 seconds. Exhale as you raise your legs, bend your knees, and roll your body sideways onto the floor, to relax.

Conditions associated with Childbirth

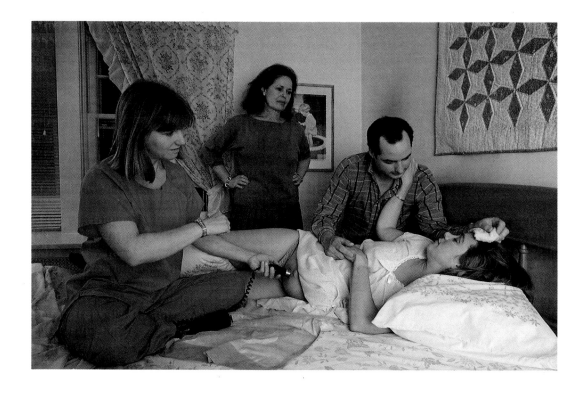

Childbirth is a momentous but exhausting event. The immense physical and emotional changes, the energy needed to make the transition, and the thrill of bringing a new life into the world, inevitably tax both mother and baby.

With improved living conditions and modern obstetric methods, childbirth now poses a minimal risk to life for most mothers and babies. But one side-effect of modern obstetric methods has been to concentrate power in the hands of hospital staff. Many women feel enormously relieved at this form of support, but some miss out on the flexibility of having their baby in natural surroundings. Gentler remedies are also more difficult to use, when the harshness of hi-technology interventional medicine interferes with the natural rhythms and responses of

The familiar surroundings and comforts of a home birth work in harmony with the gentle effects of natural medicines.

birth. Fortunately, many hospital staff nowadays are more sympathetic to the wishes of the mother and her supporters. Discuss the matter openly with your doctors and midwife, so that suitable arrangements for the type of care you want can be made in advance.

If you are unlikely to have a practitioner of natural medicine at the birth, encourage your partner or supporter to learn about remedies beforehand. She or he may have problems in concentrating while helping you through a difficult patch, so the more that is committed to memory before the event, the more effective will be the assistance.

CHILDBIRTH MEDICINE CHEST

As you prepare for labour and birth, have the following remedies ready in a handy container.

● Herbs (tincture or liquid extract): Beth root (*Trillium pendulum*), Blue cohosh (*Caulophyllum thalactroides*), and Yarrow *(Achillea millefolium)*.

● Homeopathic remedies (as pills): Arnica, Caulophyllum*, Cimcifuga*, Gelsemium*, Nux moschata, Pulsatilla*, Sepia*. The remedies marked * are suitable for almost any problem during labour and birth, as described under Treatment. They should be selected according to the normal character of the mother (see p.54).

CAUTIONS

The remedies given here are intended for you, as you approach the birth, but they are described primarily for those assisting you. During birth, you may lose your normal sense of proportion, and your emotions are very volatile. You may not be able to evaluate symptoms and signs in a logical way, or choose the right remedy.

Make sure you have the approval of your doctor or midwife, before using natural medicines. It is important to build a trusting relationship with those who will help. Air disagreements early in the pregnancy, so that you can find acceptable solutions.

REMEDIES AND EXERCISES TO HELP CHILDBIRTH

Note: See p.38 and p.54 for doses and cautions for herbal and homeopathic remedies.

Preparation for birth

● For false labour pains - Cramp bark (*Viburnum opulus*), Wild yam (*Dioscorea villosa*), or homeopathic Viburnum.

● For an insecure, restless baby - Cramp bark (*Viburnum opulus*), Wild yam (*Dioscorea villosa*), or Beth root (*Trillium pendulum*).

● For delayed labour, or if the baby goes past the due birth date - Castor oil, or one of the homeopathic remedies marked * in the panel above, matched to the mother's normal character. Consult your doctor or midwife first, then take 1 tablespoon of Castor oil, which acts on the bowels and also helps to start labour. Or take 1 homeopathic pill of 30C potency, repeated 3 days later as necessary.

During labour

A few specific treatments are mentioned here, but any of the homeopathic remedies marked * in the above panel should assist. Select one according to your constitutional character, rather than the symptoms at the time (see p.56).

● For weak contractions - Beth root (*Trillium pendulum*), 10 drops of tincture in warm water, every hour.

● For exhaustion - Yarrow (*Achillea millefolium*), half a teaspoon of tincture in warm water, every 2 hours.

● To reduce the severity of labour pains - one of the remedies marked * in the panel above.

● If you are fearful, and the fear has a known cause - homeopathic Aconite.

Continued on next page

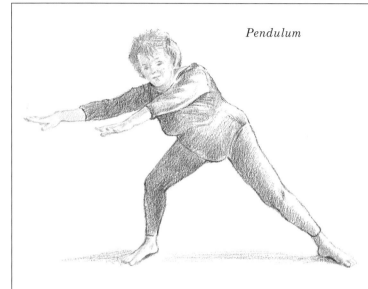

Pendulum

in front of you for balance, and your back as straight as possible. Breathe to the rhythm of your movements. Continue for as long as you like, sinking your trunk lower to open your hips.
● Swimming frog (see p.115).
● Tadpole. Lie on your back, legs straight out. Dig your elbows into the floor, your forearms perpendicular. Exhaling, raise your chest and rest your crown on the floor. If you can, after lowering your body, raise your legs off the floor with an exhalation. Inhaling, widen them apart; exhaling, bring them together again. Continue for 2-3 minutes.

Healing the perineum

The perineum may be torn at birth, or cut surgically to prevent tearing.
● Pay extra-special attention to hygiene. Regular bathing of the area, especially using a bidet, helps to prevent infection.
● A few days after the birth, take a Sitzbath 2-3 times daily. Pour into the water a tea made from 15gms (1/2ozs) of Marigold flowers (*Calendula officinalis*) and 15gms (1/2ozs) of St John's wort (*Hypericum perfoliatum*).
● Other healing herbs (taken by mouth) are Yarrow (*Achillea millefolium*) and Rosemary (*Rosmarinus officinalis*).

Continued from previous page

● For rapid, violent pains - homeopathic Aconite.
● If your mind is confused and wandering - Nux moschata.

After birth

● Homeopathic Arnica 6X, to restore balance to your nervous system. Take the first dose 3 hours after the birth, another 6 hours later, and another 12 hours after that.

Other remedies should be prescribed by a practitioner.

Exercises

Note: See p.70 for details for exercise routines. Carry out the exercises whenever you feel like it, but stop if you have any unusual pains.
● Cobbler (see p.134).
● Closed bud/Open flower. Sit on the floor with your knees out sideways, soles together, fingers interlocked behind your head. Exhaling, raise your knees toward each other and close your elbows inward in front of your face. Inhaling, lower your knees down and your elbows out as far as you can. Repeat as many times as you like.
● Squat. Just squat! Practise keeping your heels on the ground, and swing your buttocks up and down.
● Pendulum. Stand with your feet about 1 metre apart. Bending one leg, swing your trunk over to that side, straightening the other leg; then swing back. Repeat on the other side. Keep your arms hanging out

PREPARING FOR A CAESAREAN

There are times when the safest way to deliver a baby is by Caesarean section (operating on the mother and removing the baby surgically). This is a traumatic way for a baby to be delivered, but it is sometimes vital, for instance, when the placenta has grown just in front of the opening to the womb. A Caesarean is now a relatively safe operation - so much so, that many obstetricians offer it as though there were nothing unusual about it. However, many women feel afraid, and worry about this way of delivering their baby. What can be done to overcome these feelings?

The first hours and days after birth are very important in establishing the mother-baby bond. Close contact, breastfeeding, and simply being together help to develop this intensely personal link. A Caesarean delivery may interrupt this process, albeit temporarily.

Effects on the mother

The physical effects of a Caesarean on the mother are not very different from those of any other operation. In fact, she may well have an easier time than in a conventional birth, although some women feel "cheated," as though they have not really given birth at all. The absence of pain and effort, and the sudden appearance of a baby when they awake from the operation, make it seem even more dreamlike.

Bonding In a normal birth, mother and baby go through the same momentous experience together. Just as you feel close to anyone with whom you have experienced a great event, so you feel very close to your baby. If you have a Caesarean, you may feel a little distant from your baby, as though the baby is

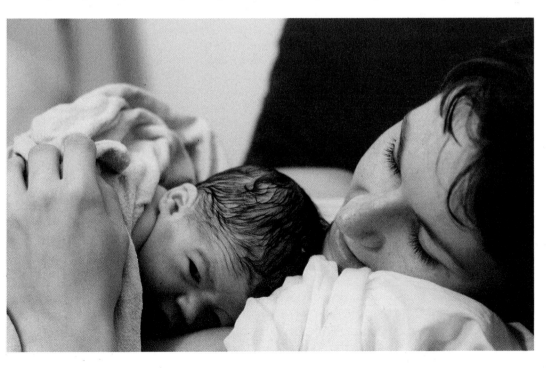

149

not really yours. This is termed "diffi-culty in bonding." The normal bond of love and attachment is not there right from the very first moment. But experi-ence has shown that in most cases, the normal bonds soon develop - usually within a week or two after the birth.

This bonding process can be speeded up if you allow time for plenty of skin contact with your baby. Spend as much time as you can with the baby close to your breast, and if possible allow your baby to go to sleep without clothes on, against your naked body. This helps to foster the primitive and wonderful connection between mother and child.

Effects on the baby

These may be more severe. In a normal birth, the baby has some choice over the time of birth, and certainly plays a large part in assisting the mother. It is clear from the rise in the baby's heart beat before the birth that she or he is keyed up and expectant, and excited about the impending and tremendous transition. The baby feels the thrill and excitement of the unknown, so that when she or he experiences the bright lights and expec-tant faces, the cold air and new skin sensations, and the strange smells - all for the first time - there is no sense of shock, but a feeling of wonder. The fact that the baby is so prepared means that she or he can go through even a quite traumatic birth without showing outward signs of shock.

A baby born by Caesarean section has received no preparation for all this. He or she may go to sleep under the influ-ence of the mother's anaesthetic, only to be rudely wakened upon coming into the world. With no preparation, the sights and sounds of the new world are thrust upon the baby. It is not surprising that many Caesarean babies show long last-ing signs of trauma and shock.

Reducing trauma and shock

There are two preparations you can make to reduce the possible negative effects of a Caesarean birth.

The medical one is the simplest: take homeopathic Arnica shortly before the operation. This will minimize the effects of physical shock.

The other preparation is to talk to the baby while he or she is still in the womb. It may seem odd to be talking to someone whom you have not yet seen, and who does not understand your language. However, there is strong evidence from "hot-house babies" in some Western countries that a baby in the womb does understand something of what its mother is trying to say.

Many mothers find that after their chil-dren are born, they instinctively know what their baby is thinking, by a sort of thought transference. This is so common, that when the second child comes, many mothers do talk to the unborn baby. In our waiting rooms, we have often seen a mother quietly talking, apparently to herself - but in reality to her unborn child. During pregnancy, instincts and forces such as thought transference come into play, which may be suppressed or forgotten in today's society.

So if a Caesarean seems inevitable, spend the days before the operation talk-ing to your baby. Explain what will happen, and that the entry into the world will appear rather sudden - but not to worry. This helps to reassure both your baby and yourself.

BREECH BIRTH

About one month before birth is due, the baby should "engage" in the mother's pelvis, taking up a position with the head down on the pelvic floor. Sometimes this does not happen, so that as birth approaches, the baby lies sideways, or with buttocks down. This is called "breech presentation." Delivery is possible this way, but the birth is more difficult and carries higher risks.

In the past, breech presentation was often remedied by the midwife or obstetrician "turning" the baby, by careful handling. Recently, this practice has become less common, because there is a risk of turning the baby with too much force and straining the umbilical cord. In many regions, the usual alternative is Caesarean delivery (see p.149) - an option many mothers wish to avoid.

There may be physical reasons why a baby cannot assume its proper head-down position. The placenta may be over or near the neck of the uterus, in the place where the baby's head should be. The umbilical cord may be too short, or wrapped around the baby's neck or limbs. Or the shape of the mother's pelvic bones may make turning difficult.

DANGER SIGNS

In rare cases, when a baby turns in the uterus it may damage the placenta, or kink the umbilical cord, or wrap the cord around its neck. The following signs indicate this type of problem. If they occur during or after the baby turns, contact your doctor or midwife at once.
- Bleeding from the uterus.
- Loss of water from the uterus.
- Contractions and labour pains.

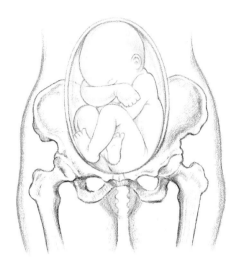

In a normal birth, the baby emerges head-first from the uterus. In a breech presentation, the baby sits the wrong way up and may be born buttocks-first.

In such cases, which can usually be diagnosed by ultrasound scanning, a Caesarean delivery is advised.

If your uterine energy is low, or if the baby lacks energy, then she or he may be too "lazy" to engage in the proper position. This is more likely if you have felt very tired during your pregnancy, but it can happen even if you are vigorous, because your unborn child's energy is the significant factor.

The emotions of anxiety and fear may contribute to breech presentation. They take energy away from the lower body - as when a sudden great fear loosens the bladder or bowels. A persistent low level of anxiety, or an acute attack of fear, can divert energy away from the lower abdomen, so that there is not enough for the baby to engage. In such cases, natural medicines can help. (Treatments for breech presentation are described on the next page.)

151

TREATMENT FOR BREECH PRESENTATION

Contact a practitioner of natural medicine for advice; in addition, inform your obstetrician or midwife. Time may be short, so try either herbs or homeopathy, plus Bach remedies, and moxibustion.

Herbs

Note: See p.38 for doses and cautions for herbs.
● The main energizing herb is Beth root (*Trillium pendulum*). Take 15 drops of tincture, 3-4 times daily.
● Raspberry leaf (*Rubus idaeus*) has similar actions, but is slower-acting.

Homeopathy

Note: See p.54 for doses and cautions for homeopathic remedies. Take the 6X potency, 3 times daily.
● If you are exhausted and you feel unable to show affection - Sepia.
● If you feel chilly and anxious - Ars. alb.
● If you are very frightened - Aconite.

Moxibustion

This simple treatment uses moxa sticks, available at health food stores or those specializing in Eastern products. If you cannot obtain moxa sticks, use a cigarette or cigar. Locate the "extreme yin" point on your little toe. Warm this with a moxa stick for 5 minutes. The treatment is usually more effective if someone else holds the moxa in their hands, as shown, and gently moves it to and fro, directing the energy from their fingers through the moxa into the extreme yin point. You should feel warmth flowing into your toe, but no burning. Repeat for the other toe. Carry out 2-3 times daily.

Bach remedies

Bach flower remedies (see p.186) are particularly helpful for feelings of fear and anxiety. Mix the remedies according to the indications given here.
● If you fear the birth itself - Mimulus.
● If you worry more about your baby's safety than your own - Red chestnut.
● If you are afraid inside, but put on a brave face - Agrimony.

Results of treatment

Within a day or two of starting treatment, you should feel the baby trying to move, although you may need to continue the remedies until the birth.

If there is a physical problem, such as a looped or taut umbilical cord, the baby is very unlikely to turn as a result of natural remedies.

Moxibustion

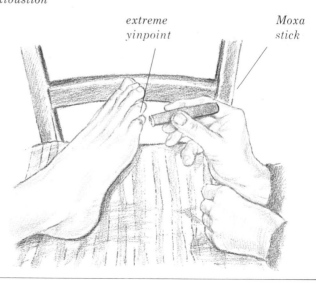

extreme
yinpoint

Moxa
stick

Postnatal Conditions

Childbirth involves a huge effort on the part of the mother. Even a relatively straightforward birth has been likened to a 30-mile run. This enormous expenditure affects the general level of energy in the lower part of your body, and also your creative energy (see p.18).

After birth, your energy levels should return to normal in a few weeks, provided you are in good health and take sufficient rest. However, you may have to return to demanding activities, such as work and looking after your family, before you have recovered your full strength. Although your general health returns, you could find that you experience various minor changes and complaints, as described here.

Loss of libido

Loss of libido, or reduced interest in sex, results from a combination of lack of creative energy, and a weakness in the lower part of the body.

Sex involves releasing large amounts of energy on different levels (see p.130), and if your total energy is low, you will probably have little interest in any activity that demands energy. This is especially common if you have to care for small children, because the great effort of childbirth is soon followed by increased demands on your creative energy, to nourish both the new baby and your other children. The advice of a practitioner is invaluable in such cases.

TREATMENT FOR LOSS OF LIBIDO

Slight loss of libido is normal after childbirth. If it is severe, consult a practitioner of natural medicine. This problem can usually be helped by natural remedies, but it is not easily treated in the home. However, exercises are of great benefit, either on their own or combined with other therapies.

Exercises

Note: See p.70 for details of exercise routines.

Natural exercise is definitely beneficial in improving sexual vitality. As well as your chosen routines, try these:

- Cobbler (see p.134).
- Half splits. Get onto all fours on the floor. Put your right leg forward, through the arch formed by your arms. Keep sliding it forward until you feel a strong therapeutic stretch behind your right knee. Raise your trunk until you feel a strong stretch on the front of your left thigh; hold this position for 30 seconds. Repeat on the other side. Then repeat for each side again. With practice you can lower your pelvic floor nearer to the ground, gradually stretching open the nerves at your sacrum, until one day you get all the way down and you are in:

- Full splits.
- Back stretch (see p.76). Like the Full splits, this stretches the nerves of your sacrum and those farther up your spine.
- Child posture. This has a similar effect to Back stretch, but is less intense, and more relaxing. Kneel, sitting on your heels. Then bend forward, keeping your buttocks on or near your heels, until your forehead touches the floor. Extend your arms beyond your head and relax for as long as you wish.
- Bow (see p.112) helps to balance the preceding exercises.

TREATMENT FOR FLABBY ABDOMEN

These two treatments, in combination, cure most cases of loose, flabby abdomen. In addition, try exercises to tone your abdominal wall.

Abdominal massage

Do the massage yourself, or ask a partner or friend to help. Rub your lower abdomen gently with the palm of the hand, in a clockwise direction, for about 5 minutes, morning and night. Aim not just to produce a pleasant physical effect, but to increase your energy level. Energy flows in abundance from the palm of the hand, and it can be directed by the thoughts and imagination of the masseur, into your abdomen. (This is why a partner or friend often has a more beneficial effect than if you self-massage.)

You may not notice much change at first, but after a few days, you should start to experience a warm, tingling feeling - a sign that energy is returning to the area.

Abdominal massage

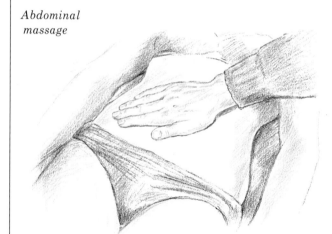

Ivy-leaf ointment

The juice of fresh ivy leaves nourishes and tones the skin. You may be able to obtain ready-made ivy-leaf ointment at a pharmacy or health store. If not, follow the instructions on p.46.

Exercises

Note: See p.70 for details of exercise routines.
● The Dynamic routine distributes energy evenly throughout your body. Add these exercises:
● Tadpole (see p.148).
● The Great pull (see p.111).

Flabby abdomen

The skin and muscular walls of your abdomen stretch enormously during pregnancy, to make room for the growing baby. After birth, the skin and muscles should contract again to their previous size, over one or two months. But if your lower abdominal energy is weak, this may not happen properly, leaving a loose and "flabby" abdomen, often with stretch marks. The two main treatments for this condition are lower abdominal massage and an ivy-leaf ointment rub.

Prolapse of the uterus

Prolapse of the uterus means a "dropping" or "falling down" of the uterus (womb). In severe cases the uterus may project outside the vagina. This is not a particularly dangerous condition, provided you do not undertake hard physical work, but it can obviously be very uncomfortable and debilitating. Natural medicines usually help, but you should first determine the cause.

Causes of uterine prolapse On the physical level, prolapse may be due to weakness of the uterine ligaments, the "stays" that hold the uterus in place. These are often strained during pregnancy and birth.

On the energy level, prolapse stems from insufficient energy in the lower part of the body. In Chinese medicine, the body's reserves of energy are stored in the lower abdomen, so that if you use up these reserves, you become more prone to prolapse. It is common for some women to experience mild uterine prolapse when they are exhausted, or when they are rushing about, trying to do too many things. In this case, you should rest, especially for an hour after your midday meal. Go to bed early. And avoid stimulants such as tea and coffee.

On the emotional level, prolapse is associated with negative feelings of helplessness and despair, and inability to complete a task without huge effort. We refer to such emotions when we say: "I've got that sinking feeling."

On the mental level, prolapse may be linked to an escapist attitude. When life is very difficult on the physical plane, you may yearn for better times and better places, or withdraw into sleep. If you spend too much time day-dreaming, and living in an imaginary world, energy tends to withdraw from your physical body. But consider: if you want to get away, where do you want to go? One of the biggest problems in "escaping" is

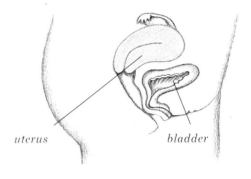

uterus   bladder

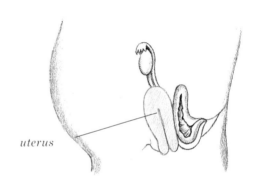

uterus

Normally, the uterus is held firmly in position above the bladder by ligaments and the general muscular tone of the abdomen (upper diagram). In prolapse, these supports become loose and the uterus slips down into the vagina (lower diagram).

that you may imagine your surroundings have changed, but you can never leave yourself behind. The desire to escape usually signifies a need to contact a higher source of energy

On the highest level, prolapse can be caused by difficulty in contacting spiritual energy. Between the ages of 40 and 50 years, the natural connection with spiritual energy reduces (see p.168), and you have to forge new links in this area. If you find it difficult to create these

TREATMENT FOR PROLAPSE OF THE UTERUS

There are several orthodox treatments for uterine prolapse. These include inserting a rubber ring inside the vagina, to hold up the uterus; minor surgery to "hitch up" the ligaments, or hysterectomy (see p.174).

Many cases of prolapse respond well to natural medicine, particularly acupuncture. Other useful therapies include osteopathy, homeopathy, and herbs. But it is wise to consult a practitioner.

Herbs

Note: See p.38 for doses and cautions for herbs.
● False unicorn root (*Chamaelirium luteum*) and True unicorn root (*Aletris farinosa*) strengthen the pelvic region.
● If Unicorn roots are not available, try Water lily (*Nymphaea alba*).
● Black cohosh (*Cimicifuga racemosa*) is a tonic to the reproductive system, and complements Unicorn roots.
● White poplar (*Populus tremuloides)* moves the energy in the lower bowels. Add it to the other herbs.

Exercises

Note: See p.70 for details of exercise routines.
● The Dynamic routine powerfully rectifies the polarity of energy in your body, which causes the prolapse. In addition:
● Neckstand (see p.77).
● Plough (see p.77).
● Topsy-turvy. Sit "the wrong way round" on a sofa or large armchair: bottom up against the backrest, back lying on the seat, head and arms dangling behind you to the floor. Now just relax. Stay there as long as you like. This "non-exercise" can be profoundly restful, since it nourishes your pituitary and pineal glands. After, lie flat on the floor to let your blood redistribute evenly.

Point therapy

Prolapse is often associated with loss of energy through the top of the head. This can sometimes be remedied by gently massaging the head. A Chinese folk remedy is to put a crushed castor-oil bean on the vertex of the skull and massage this gently into the scalp.

Homeopathy

Note: See p.54 for doses and cautions for homeopathic remedies.
The most effective method is constitutional prescribing at high potencies. If possible, consult a homeopath. If not, consult the Materia medica (see pp.57-69), paying attention to the dynamic features. The following may help: Sepia, Calc. carb., Helonias, Podophyllum, Pulsatilla, Nat. mur., or Stannum.

Progress of treatment

If uterine prolapse is treated in the early stages, you should see improvement in a week or so - not necessarily in the symptoms, but in your general mood and optimism. Long-standing cases require prolonged treatment, and your symptoms and mood may worsen at first.

Point therapy massage

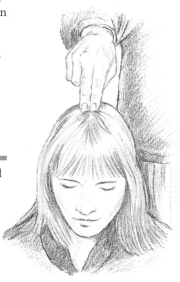

TREATMENT FOR STRESS INCONTINENCE

Herbs

Note: See p.38 for doses and cautions for herbs.

The following herbs strengthen the lower body:
- Beth root (*Trillium pendulum*).
- False unicorn root (*Chamaelirium luteum*).
- True unicorn root (*Aletris farinosa*).

Herbs which tighten and dry loose tissues include:
- Sweet sumach (*Rhus aromatica*).
- Cranesbill (*Geranium maculatum*).
- A home prescription is Beth root (*Trillium pendulum*), Cranesbill (*Geranium maculatum*), and Sweet sumach (*Rhus aromatica*). Mix equal quantities of the tinctures of each, and take 30 drops of the mixture in warm water, up to 3 times daily.

Together, these herbs have a local effect, toning and tightening the urogenital area. They should help, provided your overall energy level is good. If it is weak, correct this first. Also, if you are overweight, tackling this at the same time will make the herbs more effective.

Homeopathy

Note: See p.54 for doses and cautions for homeopathic remedies.
- If you have a slight soreness in the bladder, and you feel you may not really want to enter into the role of being a mother - Causticum.
- If you have a tendency to being "hot-headed" and very sensitive to external events - Ferr. phos.
- If you experience lots of watery discharges, and you feel negative about life, even to the point of depression - Nat. mur.
- If your moods fluctuate, so that you swing from sunny optimism to tearful worry and back - Pulsatilla.
- If you are sensitive to noise, forgetful, and tend to twitch a lot - Zincum metallicum.

Exercises

Note: See p.70 for details of exercise routines.
- Weak routine, graduating to Dynamic routine. Add:
- Pelvic energizer (see p.104).
- The Great pull (see p.111).

---

links, you may not receive enough spiritual energy to provide the inspiration and fire in your life, which then seems flat and dull. This is a common cause for overall lack of energy. We refer to it as "head in the clouds," where we instinctively reach upward, yet cannot find the true energy source. In this case, take life more calmly; leave time for reflection.

Stress incontinence

Stress incontinence means involuntary passing of a small amount of urine, during or just after some sudden physical stress, such as coughing, laughing, or jumping. A recent survey revealed that about one-third of all women over 40 years of age experience this problem at some time.

This type of incontinence is due partly to insufficient energy in the lower part of the body, especially the pelvic region. Like the conditions mentioned previously, it is often a combination of weak physical energy, and weak or undirected creative energy (see p.18). Natural medicines can help, but it is usually necessary to visit a practitioner, for more satisfactory results.

POSTNATAL (POSTPARTUM) DEPRESSION

Almost all new mothers suffer from a degree of depression after childbirth, even if only for a few hours or days. In some cases, feelings deepen to despair, which can persist for months.

The symptoms of PND/PPD are mainly on the emotional level. As a new mother, you may feel engulfed by an emotional black wave, which has smothered your usual stability and resilience. The underlying cause is nearly always lack of energy, so that even a small problem takes more energy than you have.

Lack of physical energy The tremendous efforts of childbirth deplete your energy reserves on all levels. You are more likely to succumb to depression if you tend to "weak" patterns of illness (see p.98), or if the birth was very difficult.

A contributing factor is being unable to take sufficient rest after childbirth. In the first few days, there may be an overwhelming sense of euphoria. This stems partly from the joy at having successfully brought your baby into the world, but it also has a hormonal complement. It means that you do not feel tired, even though you really are, and so you may not rest as much as you should. Soon, your reserves of energy have gone, and the hormonal effect wears off. You may then come down with a terrific "bump."

Emotional factors Although the primary cause of PND/PPD is on the energy level, certain emotions aggravate the situation. You may feel guilty that you do not love your baby enough, or you may have problems in bonding (see p.149). Normally, you would soon recognize and tackle such feelings. But in your depleted state, they bring on sensations of inadequacy. Some mothers enter a

vicious circle, in which they feel they are failing the new baby by being depressed, which brings on greater hopelessness, and makes things worse.

Willpower The creative energy so important in childbirth is linked to willpower (see p.18). After the birth, your creative energy is low, which leaves very little willpower. As a result, you lack your usual resolve to "snap out of it," feeling there is no point in recovery.

A new mother may even believe that utter hopelessness is natural. She feels worse than ever, yet trying to change things seems futile. In such cases, it is vital that the people around should lend encouragement, helping her to select the remedies and take positive steps.

Avoiding PND/PPD

● Before the birth, take care to build up energy reserves (see p.127), and consider mineral and vitamin supplements.
● After the birth, if you have difficulty in sleeping or feel over-excited, try a proprietary herbal sleeping tablet. Or make a sleeping mixture of Passion flower (*Passiflora incarnata*), Valerian (*Valeriana officinalis*), and Wild lettuce (*Lactuta virosa*). Take 30 drops of the mixture of tinctures, in water, before going to bed. These herbs are very safe, and may be taken up to eight times in 24 hours. Besides helping you to sleep, they will also calm your baby if you are breastfeeding. If possible, check with a qualified practitioner before starting self-treatment.
● If your appetite is poor, try Gentian (*Gentiana lutea*) and Berberis (*Berberis officinale*), 20 drops of the mixture of tinctures, in water before each meal.

158

TREATMENT FOR POSTNATAL (POSTPARTUM) DEPRESSION

Herbs

Note: See p.38 for doses and cautions for herbs.

If possible, check with a qualified practitioner before you begin self-treatment.
- Yarrow (*Achillea millefolium*), Hawthorn (*Crataegus oxycantha*), and Licorice (*Glycyrrhiza glabra*). Place 1 level 5mls teaspoon of each herb in a non-metallic or non-stick pan and add about 200mls (1/3pint) of water. Briefly bring to the boil. When still warm, strain and drink. Take 3 times daily.

Homeopathy

Note: See p.54 for doses and cautions for homeopathic remedies.
- The remedy of choice is Platinum. If this does not help after a few days, select one of the following.
- If your life seems joyless, and those around you do not appear to give support - Sepia.
- If you are despairing, and also harbour vindictive feelings - Nit. ac.
- If you are very apathetic, and you lost much blood during the birth - China.
- If you are constantly weepy, but without obvious cause - Apis. mel.
- If you cannot sleep soundly - Lilium tig.

Bach remedies

(See p.186 for information on Bach remedies.)
- If you feel nothing will lift the depression - Gorse.
- If you feel great anguish - Sweet chestnut.
- If you are suddenly struck by deep melancholy for no obvious reason - Mustard.

Exercises

Note: See p.70 for details of exercise routines.
- Easy routine, merging into Dynamic routine.
- If you feel apathetic about even the slightest exertion, the Weak routine is a saving standby.
- You may view formal exercise routines as requiring too much willpower. Instead, take a gentle stroll in the fresh air, to get your energy circulating again.
- However bad you feel, at least do something. Even a couple of exercises daily can put a silver lining on the cloud. Try doing these four in order:
- Child posture (see p.153).
- Hug. Stand with your feet about shoulder-width apart. Cross your arms over your chest and hold your shoulders. Breathing out, gently and slowly swing your trunk round to one side, coming up on the toes of the opposite foot. Remain like this for a few breaths. Breathing in, face the front again, then repeat on the other side. Change the crossing of your arms, and do the whole exercise again on both sides.
- Hillock. Lay a cushion or two on the floor. Then lie your back on top of them, letting your head and buttocks dangle down at either end. Relax like this for a few minutes.
- Topsy-turvy (see p.156).

Hug

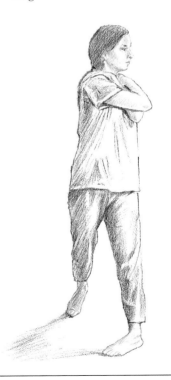

BREASTFEEDING PROBLEMS

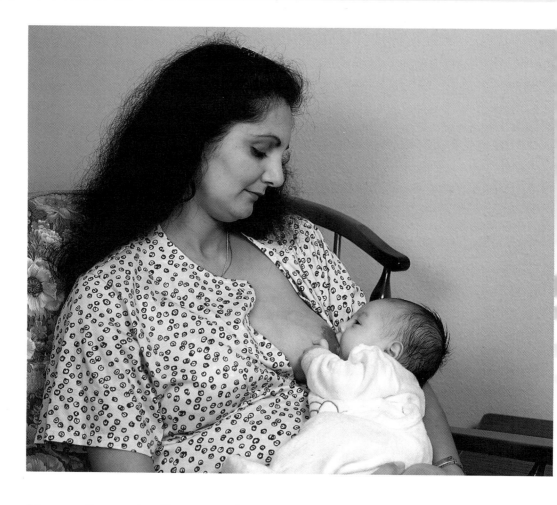

Many mothers naturally want to breast-feed their babies. They feel that breast-feeding is the best way to give the baby its first food. Breast milk is a composite, living substance that provides complete nourishment, and gives the best defense against disease. However, several types of problems can arise.

In fact, breastfeeding is by no means always easy. Although it is a natural human function, our society has changed so much that breastfeeding, along with other aspects of childrearing (like toilet-training), is an unfamiliar sight. It has to

Breastfeeding provides the baby with a complete, natural food. It is also an important part of developing the priceless bond between mother and baby.

be taught. Societies with a more natural, down-to-earth approach to childcare view breastfeeding as a common, every-day event. Mothers freely feed their babies in public. In many Western situations, mothers feel that they must feed their babies in private. This strained social attitude contributes to some of the problems that surround breastfeeding.

As a new mother, your reaction upon encountering problems may be: "Why me? It seems so easy for everyone else!" Yet surveys show that very few women have no problems in breastfeeding. Most are minor: the baby falls asleep during a feed, or burping (winding) is awkward. Some problems are more severe; in these situations, natural medicine can help.

How breast milk is produced

Orthodox medicine and natural medicine take different views about the way milk is produced. However, the views are

The body's "master gland" is the tiny pituitary, at the base of the brain. Through its close connections with the hypothalamus, it links emotional states to hormone levels.

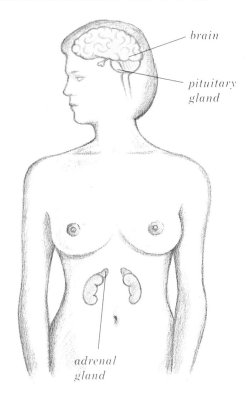

brain

pituitary gland

adrenal gland

FOODS THAT AFFECT BREAST MILK SUPPLY

Foods that increase milk supply
- Brewer's yeast, stout (mild) beers.
- Pine kernels.
- Lettuce.
- Boiled turnips, boiled radish.

Foods that decrease milk supply
Foods that diminish the supply of milk are usually a disadvantage when breastfeeding, but they can be useful if you have too much milk - for example, when weaning.
- Lentils.
- Celery leaves.
- Certain herbs, including Sage, Rue, Parsley, Basil, and Periwinkle.

---

complementary, and help to give further understanding of causes and treatments.

In the view of orthodox medicine, the milk glands are specialized forms of sweat glands. Just as the sweat glands produce a mixture of salts and fats, in perspiration, so the milk glands produce a refined form of milk and salts.

Sweat glands also produce different compositions of perspiration depending on your mood. The "cold sweat" of fear has very different ingredients from the watery perspiration of a hot summer's day. Similarly, the nature of breast milk varies according to your mood. Even a relatively small change of mood and emotions can soon produce a large change in milk composition.

These changes occur because the secretion of milk is controlled by hormones, which are in turn controlled by the pituitary gland, the small but powerful

161

CAUTION

Some of the ingredients in foods you eat pass into your breast milk, and will be taken in by your baby. They include the active components of certain herbs and other natural remedies. The treatments advised here are exceptionally safe, and have been used by breastfeeding mothers through the ages.

However, before you start self-treatment, consult a herbalist or practitioner of natural medicine. There may be unforeseen side-effects, or you or your baby might develop a sensitivity or allergy.

If you suspect an allergy, keep a food diary of your own meals, and include your baby's responses. You could find a link between a food you eat, and the baby's reactions a few hours or days later.

"master gland" located just under the brain. The pituitary has intimate links with the hypothalamus, the part of the brain above, which deals with emotions and feelings. So, from the higher centres of the brain, through the hypothalamus, the pituitary, and the hormonal glands such as the adrenals, your mental and emotional state is connected to your hormonal and physical reactions.

The viewpoint of Chinese medicine is that milk is transformed blood. It is said that ten drops of blood are needed to make one drop of milk. This is not meant literally - blood is not converted directly into milk. Nevertheless, there is a close relationship between the strength and composition of blood and the quantity and quality of breast milk.

If you are generally healthy, with good reserves of energy, you should be able to produce sufficient milk without becoming anaemic. But if you exhaust your energy supply, or eat poor-quality food, or if your baby is particularly demanding, your blood will become depleted, and so will your breast milk.

Emotional factors Childbirth takes huge amounts of energy, and may leave you emotionally drained. In this state, you are prone to over-react; little problems become big ones, and big problems seem insuperable. If your new baby is tiresome and taxing, you may find yourself becoming agitated and almost hysterical - quite unlike your usual self. You may also feel that family and friends are not lending enough support.

These reactions are common soon after the birth. They may affect your milk temporarily, but the supply should return with your energy and stability. Therefore, do not necessarily rush to the natural medicine chest. In the week or so after the birth, rest is the best treatment. If problems still persist, try the remedies advised here.

As you settle into your new role, any factor that obstructs the natural flow of love for your baby is also likely to affect your milk supply, through the hormonal and emotional links described above. You may find, like many mothers, that loving your baby is not always easy. You may have mixed feelings: although you love her or him in a way you could not have imagined, at the same time any baby can be tiresome and obstinate. It is quite possible to feel love and hate simultaneously. Such conflicting feelings not only cause distress, but they also affect breast milk supply.

Milk obstruction and milk fever

Milk which gets obstructed or blocked in the breasts is a common problem. It may happen because you produce more milk than your baby can take, or because the milk is too thick, or your energy is not circulating well.

If congestion in the breasts persists, the milk may become infected and go "sour," giving rise to the problem known as milk fever. This is characterized by high fever and engorged breasts, and is potentially quite dangerous. Rapid treatment by antibiotic drugs has much reduced its risks; but this condition also responds to natural medicines.

Principles of treatment In the view of natural medicine, the principles of treatment for milk fever are similar to those for an ordinary fever. They are: to clear excess heat from your body by encouraging perspiration; and to clear congestion of

---

TREATMENT FOR MILK OBSTRUCTION AND MILK FEVER

Herbs

Note: See p.38 for doses and cautions for herbs.
● Herbs that relieve congestion in the breasts include Cleavers (*Galium aparine*), Poke root (*Phytolacca decandra*), Wormwood (*Artemisia absinthum*), and Hawthorn (*Crataegus oxycantha*).
● Herbs which help to open the skin pores, to allow perspiration and clear fever, are Yarrow (*Achillea millefolium*), Elderflower (*Sambucus nigra*), Peppermint (*Mentha piperata*), and Catmint (*Nepeta cataria*).
● A suitable home prescription is Cleavers, Yarrow, and Hawthorn, standard dose of each. If possible, prepare the herbs as a tea, rather than tinctures. Take 1 cup of tea every hour until you start to perspire, then drink 1 cup every 2-3 hours.
● If there is pus formation, add Echinacea (*Echinacea purpurea*).

External treatment

Make a strong tea of Cleavers (*Galium aparine*) and Catmint (*Nepeta cataria*), with about 25gms (1oz) of each dried herb in the cupful of water. When the tea has cooled to body temperature, strain off the herbs, soak a small cloth in the liquid, and apply it to the affected area. Rinse the cloth, re-soak and reapply it, every 15 minutes.

Homeopathy

Note: See p.54 for doses and cautions for homeopathic remedies.
● The remedy of choice is Phytolacca. Take 1 dose of 6X potency hourly until you notice some improvement. Then take 1 dose every 4 hours, alternating with one of the following remedies as indicated.
● If you have alternating fever and chills, and you feel frightened - Aconite.
● If you have a high fever, with a red face, perspiration, and bursting headache - Belladonna.
● If your fever is accompanied by fluid retention - Apis mel.
For congestion in the breast:
● If there is pus formation - Silica and Calc. sulph.
● If the congestion is due to injury - Bellis or Arnica.
● If you experience neuralgic pains in the breast, possibly due to an old injury - Conium.
● If you have strong, tight pains in the breast, but no redness - Bryonia.

163

fluids, in this case by getting the energy moving and circulating to the breasts, in order to disperse congested milk.

Orthodox medical treatment is to administer an antibiotic drug, that kills the invading bacteria causing the fever. But this may well destroy some of the beneficial qualities of the milk, and reduce the baby's natural immunity. And although the antibiotic clears the inflammation and removes immediate risks to health, it does not improve your energy circulation, and therefore fails to strike at the root of the condition. The difference between the orthodox and natural approaches is summed up by this (freely-translated) Chinese saying, when there is an unwanted person present: "No need to kill the guest - simply open the door."

Symptoms and general advice Regard soreness, swelling, and tenderness in the breast as warning signs. Take prompt action, to avoid further complications.
● The main advice, given repeatedly in this book, is that "rest is best." This is especially important in the first weeks after childbirth.
● Avoid stimulants such as tea and coffee. Instead, take relaxants such as a Chamomile (*Anthemis nobilis*) or Valerian (*Valeriana officinalis*) herbal tea.
● Eat light foods only, avoiding rich or heavy meals.
● Try to spread some of your workload. Enlist a helper for your other children, or ask for the aid of colleagues at work.

Cracked and sore nipples

Sore nipples are very common, especially when you start to breastfeed. You can apply a proprietary ointment (often based on the herb Chamomile), but some-times this is not enough. In severe cases, the soreness and dryness makes the skin on your nipples cracked and fissured, with great pain when the baby suckles.

In the view of natural medicine, sore or cracked nipples are due to the same condition which causes soreness elsewhere in the skin: weak blood. There is insufficient blood to nourish the skin, which becomes dry and sore when exposed to repeated suckling. Treat as for anaemia (see p.93), plus the remedies listed opposite.

Insufficient milk

Some mothers who want to breastfeed find that they do not have enough milk. This is a problem particularly when the baby is short of energy, because she or he does not suckle strongly, and a strong sucking action stimulates milk secretion. A common reaction is to give the baby extra feeds from a bottle. But the baby is then less hungry, and does not have to suck at the bottle quite so hard. So she or he gradually becomes more lazy, and your milk supply decreases further.

Counteract this problem in several ways. First, consult your physician or health adviser about breastfeeding. Often, an apparent lack of milk stems from the baby not latching onto the nipple properly, and therefore not sucking effectively. A breast pump can help stimulate milk production. (Treatments are listed on p.166.)

Indigestible milk

Your baby may seem unable to digest your milk properly, showing symptoms of nausea or vomiting, or abdominal pain and colic. The problem is rarely physical.

TREATMENT FOR CRACKED AND SORE NIPPLES

General care

- Expose your breasts to air and sunlight as much as possible.
- Apply ice packs to your nipples for a few minutes before and after feeds.
- Rub in some Olive oil, Lanolin, Almond oil, or Comfrey root ointment.
- Massage Aloe vera ointment into the nipples, to reduce inflammation. Do this after feeds, since it has a bitter taste.

The above remedies are safe for the baby to take. The oils are nourishing, and Aloe vera is a tonic for his or her stomach.

Herbs

Choose herbal remedies as for anaemia (see p.93). If in doubt, treat as for the weak pattern of anaemia.

Homeopathy

Note: See p.54 for doses and cautions for homeopathic remedies.

- Sepia is the main remedy.
- If your nipples are very sore and you experience pain as the baby sucks - Phytolacca.
- If your nipples are blistered - Graphites.
- If your nipples are very cracked and deeply fissured - Silica.
- If your nipples are sore, but with few cracks - Causticum.
- If your nipples are chapped and "frayed" in appearance - Sulphur.

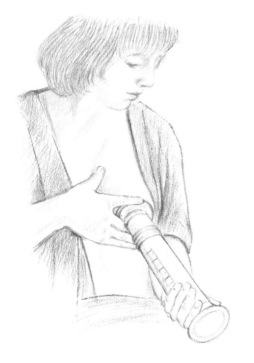

It normally occurs at the vital and emotional levels (see p.15), because your energy reserves - or those of the baby - are unbalanced or depleted. The main patterns are "thin milk" and "mismatched milk," as described below.

"Thin milk" pattern   When your own energy and vitality are running low, your milk may become thin and watery. The strength of your blood is not sufficient to produce fully nourishing milk. Typical symptoms of this pattern in the mother are:

- you are tired all the time,
- you feel overburdened and find it difficult to cope, and
- you may be thin, with a pale face.

Milk production relies partly on stimulation of the nipple by the baby's sucking movements. Use of a breast pump helps to mimic this stimulation and maintain milk production.

165

The baby gains weight slowly, if at all, and she or he brings up a little milk ("posseting") just after feeding.

"Mismatched milk" pattern If your liver is out of balance, it cannot metabolize the milk's constituents correctly. This is often due to stress, and may happen if you have strong, active attitudes and do demanding, creative work. Part of the treatment is to slow down and reduce tensions in your life, especially while you are breastfeeding.

Or the milk is mismatched because your own constitutional type is quite different from your baby's. For example, you may be vigorous and robust, while your baby is quiet and delicate.

Typical symptoms in the mother are:
■ you feel physically tense,
■ you are easily irritated by your baby,
■ you may have some indigestion, and
■ you feel better after alcohol.

The baby rejects the milk and "pulls faces," and brings up curdled milk, usually some time after the feed. She or

---

TREATMENT FOR INSUFFICIENT MILK

General advice

● Above all, take enough rest. If your nights are troubled, relax during the daytime.
● Self-care for insufficient milk is the same as for anaemia (see p.93).
● Eat nourishing, high-vitality foods (see p.29).

Herbs

Note: See p.38 for doses and cautions for herbs.
● Among the many herbs which help to increase milk production are Goat's rue (*Galega officinalis*), Dill seed (*Anethum graveolens*), Fennel (*Foeniculum vulgare*), Aniseed (*Anisum pimpinella*), Holy thistle (*Carduus benedictus*), Milk thistle (*Carduus marianus*), Fenugreek (*Trigonella foenum-graecum*), Vervain

(*Verbena officinalis*), and Nettle (*Urtica dioica*).

Choose 2-3 herbs which have agreeable flavours, and take the standard dose, preferably as a tea, 3 or more times daily.

Homeopathy

Note: See p.54 for doses and cautions for homeopathic remedies.

Take 1 dose of 6X potency, 3 times daily, until the milk supply resumes.
● If your moods are changeable - Pulsatilla.
● If you are inwardly depressed, but put on a brave face for others - Nat. mur.
● If the milk supply reduces after you have been greatly excited - 1 dose of Ignatia, at 30C potency.
● If you feel very exposed and sensitive - Asafoetida.

● If the milk supply reduces after a cold or a bout of influenza - Sulphur.

Exercises

Note: See p.70 for details of exercise routines.

Keeping an open flow through the energy channel relating to the stomach is helpful in breastfeeding. Do any one exercise from each of the following three groups (for page numbers, see the Index on p.188):
● Start with Camel, Laid back, Hillock, Corner hang, or Bow.
● Follow with Temple guardian, Film director, or Mermaid.
● And then Back stretch, Forward stretch, or Leg stretch.
● Finally, relax.

TREATMENT FOR INDIGESTIBLE MILK

Herbs

Note: See p.38 for doses and cautions for herbs. Prepare a herb tea, rather than taking the tincture.
● For the thin milk pattern, herbal remedies are the same as for the weak energy pattern of anaemia (see p.98). The following are particularly useful: Fennel seed (*Foeniculum vulgare*), Licorice (*Glycyrrhiza glabra*), Yarrow (*Achillea millefolium*), and Hawthorn (*Crataegus oxycantha*).
● For the mismatched milk pattern, try Fringe tree (*Chionanthus virginica*), Valerian (*Valeriana officinalis*), and Hawthorn (*Crataegus oxycantha*).

● If you find fatty foods difficult to digest, add Black root (*Leptandra virginica*) to the above prescription.

Homeopathy

Note: See p.54 for doses and cautions for homeopathic remedies.
For the thin milk pattern:
● If you are thin and pale-faced - Silica.
● If you feel washed out and "grey," and you lack support - Sepia.
● If you have become rather fat and flabby, and you have a tendency to constipation - Calc. carb.
● If you cry easily, but the tears are usually short-lived - Pulsatilla.

For the mismatched milk pattern:
● If your milk seems incompatible with your baby's digestion, but there are no obvious symptoms - Aethusa.
● If you feel angry and nauseous - Nux vomica.
● If you are irritable, easily become very angry, and suffer muscular tensions and cramps - Chamomilla.
● If you have become rather flabby - Calc. carb.
● If you are thin and pale-faced - Silica.
● If your milk seems too rich, and you dislike fatty foods - Pulsatilla.

he may also grimace or even cry loudly from abdominal pain, and there are green or runny bowel motions.

General advice when breastfeeding

● Remember that there are two ways to treat indigestible milk problems. You can give natural medicine to the baby, so that her or his digestion is strengthened (check with your practitioner first). Or as the Chinese say, you can "treat the mother to treat the child."
● Try to look after yourself, and your own mental state, as well as your baby. Do something that you enjoy, since if you feel better, so will your baby.

● Try to get rid of guilt feelings. The situation is not "your fault," it occurs naturally and is very common. Equally, try to admit your feelings to yourself. If you are cross and irritable with your week-old baby, do not pretend otherwise.
● When your baby first arrives, you may believe that you should love her or him all the time. It can be distressing to find yourself feeling angry towards such a small and vulnerable creature, but it does happen - especially when the baby rejects your milk, seeming also to reject the love that goes with it. This is a natural reaction, but persevere. It may help to talk to mothers with older children, about how they overcame the problem.

Conditions associated with the Menopause

Technically, the menopause is the last menstrual period. In everyday language, this term also covers the time when the menstrual cycle gradually ceases, and with it ovulation (and fertility). In most women, this occurs between 48 and 54 years of age, but there is wide variation.

This important stage of life is rarely talked about openly. The most you may know about it, before you experience it yourself, is that you may have a bad time! This extraordinary attitude to a natural change is partly a leftover from the days when women's problems were rarely discussed in public. It is also due to the nature of the change itself, which is complex and deeply personal.

In traditional medicine, the menopause is viewed as one of life's "gateways" (see p.21). The role of natural remedies at this time is to open the gate; it is up to you to take the opportunity, and walk through.

The role of spiritual energy During your childbearing years, you have a cyclical contact with spiritual energy, which enables you to conceive and bear children (see p.88). At the menopause, this connection gradually weakens, and you no longer have a reliable input of spiritual energy. As a result, you generally have less energy available to give to others. Natural medicines can help you make contact with your spiritual energy.

In previous years, you may have spent your own creative energy on your family and/or career, or caring for relatives, or some equally taxing task. After the menopause, you can no longer donate energy freely without becoming depleted. For perhaps the first time, you have to learn to put yourself first. This entails changing the way you relate to your family, friends, and work colleagues. You may feel selfish and guilty about concentrating on your own needs. And there may be resistance to your changing attitudes, from the rest of your family and those at work.

Social factors In the West, youth and beauty are often valued more than old age - a concept reinforced by advertising and media events. This notion is rarely balanced by images of the wisdom and tranquility that age and experience foster. Small wonder, then, many women feel anxious about approaching the menopause. As their youthful beauty fades, they are apprehensive about a loss of standing in society.

Interestingly, in cultures where older women gain increased status by becoming the head of the family, menopausal problems are much less common. This contrast indicates that factors other than hormonal changes are involved.

Periods during the menopause

The menopause shows itself in one of several ways. Your periods may gradually become more scanty over many months until they disappear; they may cease altogether within a few cycles; they may vary from heavy to light, but gradually reduce; or the intervals between them may increase to several months, until the expected last period never comes. Many women find that their monthly body rhythm continues for some years after their actual periods

Regard the menopause not as the start of increasing limitations, but as the time when you can take up those interests which you have always wanted to pursue.

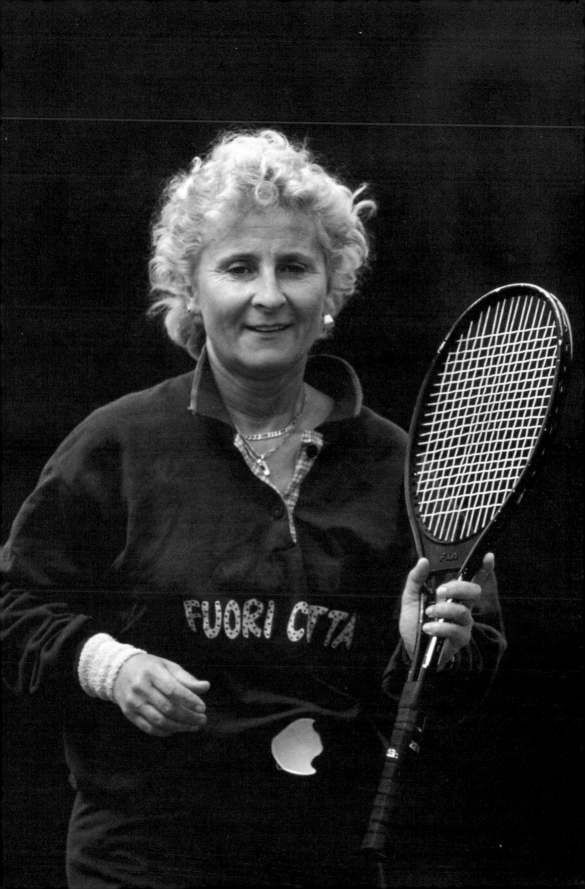

HORMONE REPLACEMENT THERAPY (HRT)

Female hormone levels decline as you go through the menopause. An orthodox medical treatment is to administer a "replacement" hormone dose, to maintain their high levels artificially. This may temporarily relieve severe menopausal symptoms.

In natural medicine, the diminishing hormone levels are seen not so much as the cause of problems, but as a sign of more fundamental changes. The real needs are to establish new lines of energy flow in your body, to contact the power of spiritual energy (see p.14), and to find a truly satisfying occupation or activity.

---

stop. The ovaries continue to secrete hormones on the same pattern, but at insufficient strength for periods to occur. However, signs such as PMS (PMT) may persist (see p.90).

Preparing for the menopause

If you have difficult periods, you may look forward to being free from monthly discomfort. Instinctively, you realize that the menopause offers great opportunity. On the other hand, if you have previously enjoyed excellent health, you may view the transition with concern. In either case, if you nurture a positive attitude, you are more likely to experience a smooth transition.

A positive approach First, think about the changes the menopause may bring, and how you might capitalize on them. For some women, this stage of life is a time of increasing freedom. The children are at school, or have left home, and they are usually less demanding than when young. You may have a measure of financial security, and an established career. For the first time in many years, you have the time and energy to do what you want. A natural reaction is to start a new project, redeploying the energy you once used to bring up a family or carve out a career.

For women who started a family in their late thirties or early forties, the menopause can come at a time when they are still directing much energy into childcare, thereby increasing demands. Part of the answer is to recognize the situation, and enlist help.

The creative urge A compulsive urge to be active and creative is characteristic of the menopausal transition. This signifies your need to build up a spiritual connection, and to express your true inner self.

Your new activity or occupation should provide the means for spiritual reconnection and for building new relationships. If you keep these five thoughts in mind, the time of the menopause should encourage your awareness and wisdom to unfold:
● Start an activity that will refresh and invigorate you, and bring calm and joy - not one that will exhaust you.
● Focus on the joy of a pastime, career, or occupation, rather than the material achievements or results.
● Concentrate on the cool stillness in your life (see p.18).
● Develop activities which express what your innermost self wants to do.
● Remember that this is the time of life to put yourself first.

HOT FLUSHES (HOT FLASHES)

These are perhaps the commonest of menopausal symptoms in our Western society. They may pass so fleetingly that you hardly notice them, or they may be severe enough to bring great embarrassment and near-incapacitation.

Symptoms

In a typical case, you first experience a sudden rush of heat - especially to the head, but often through your whole body. You begin to perspire, your heart thumps or flutters (palpitations), and you feel extremely uncomfortable. The perspiration can be so severe that you are rapidly

drenched in sweat. After a few minutes the heat starts to subside, and you gradually begin to feel normal again.

Hot flushes (also called hot flashes) may happen once every few days, or more than 30 times daily. When they occur frequently, they can cause great fatigue, and even force you to take bed rest.

Causes and factors

In orthodox medicine, this condition result from a combination of vasomotor instability and hormonal imbalance. Vasomotor instability is an unpredictable pattern of blood vessel dilation due to erratic nerve control of the blood vessels, which may be influenced by the fluctuating hormone levels. Hormonal imbalance affects the adrenal glands (see p.161), making them release a sudden surge of adrenaline. This is the "fight or flight" hormone that prepares the body for physical exertion in an emergency, and one of its effects is to dilate (widen) certain blood vessels.

In Chinese medicine, the causes of hot flushes (hot flashes) are twofold. One is the normal reduction during the menopause of "water energy," the other is accumulated "excess heat." It is said that as the water energy declines, it is no longer sufficient to damp down the excess heat, which flares up.

Decline of water energy The menopause brings a natural decline in your water energy, which is closely related to the still, quiet centre of your spiritual energy (see p.15). In the same way that water is stored in reservoirs, so water energy is related to your overall energy reserves. If you continually draw on your reserves, through overwork, or late

---

MOOD SWINGS AND DEPRESSION

"Mood swings," when emotions run out of control, are common symptoms of the menopause. You may overreact, as you rage at a comparatively minor irritation one minute, then laugh wildly at nothing in particular the next. These actions are due to energy changes, in particular, a lack of water energy. Sometimes menopausal mood swings are not so much between laughter and sadness, as between sadness and black despair. The problem usually stems from difficulty in finding out what you really want, and responding to that need.

The treatments described here can help to even out mood problems. Difficulties in finding your sense of self-worth and recognizing your innermost desires run deeper, and need to be tackled in a different way, often by sympathetic counselling.

171

TREATMENT FOR HOT FLUSHES (HOT FLASHES)

Herbs

Note: See p.38 for doses and cautions for herbs.
- Suitable herbs include Chaste tree (*Vitex agnus-castus*), Yarrow (*Achillea millefolium*), Wormwood (*Artemisia absinthum*), Lady's slipper (*Cypripedium pubescens*), or Mistletoe (*Viscum album*).

Take the standard dose, 3 times daily, diluted in water.

Continue these herbs for up to a year if necessary.

Homeopathy

Note: See p.54 for doses and cautions for homeopathic remedies.
- If you are timid and indecisive - Graphites.
- If you cannot identify what you really desire, and you cover this by compulsively talking too much - Lachesis.
- If you cannot stop over-working - Phosphorus.
- If you drive yourself too hard in all aspects of life - Nux vomica.

Consult the Materia medica (see pp.57-69) to decide on the most appropriate remedy. The high potencies often needed are best taken under the advice of a practitioner.

Exercises

See the exercise routines on pp.72-81. Regular exercise, breathing, and meditation can replace other life rhythms which fade at this time. Choose the routine you like best; do it daily.

---

nights, or taxing your digestion through unsuitable food, your reserves of energy will gradually decrease. The frequency and severity of hot flushes (hot flashes) then increase.

Emotional factors Water energy can be exhausted if you do something which, deep inside, you know is against your will. During the childbearing years, a constant supply of spiritual energy maintains your water energy, enabling you to continue to enjoy life while still devoting so much energy to supporting others.

At the menopause, as your spiritual energy fades, you are thrown back onto your own resources. At this time, if you are still involved in activities which you truly want to abandon, you cannot draw on your energy reserves, and your water energy runs out. The solution is to recognize your real desires, and thus take appropriate action.

Spiritual factors Water energy declines when you lack contact with the quiet, still energy that is the source of life. As the natural supply of still energy reduces with age, it can be sapped by an excessively busy, active life. Try to set aside "quality quiet-time" to clear your mind of day-to-day preoccupations.

Some women turn to religion or other spiritual involvement, as a way of replenishing their energies.

Accumulation of "heat" Too much heat in the body can have dietary causes, as explained on p.30. A healthy eating pattern does much to eliminate the problem of hot flushes (hot flashes), as does physical exercise.

On the emotional level, heat is generated by the "hot" feelings of anger, resentment, bitterness, and frustration. It is also created by continually pushing the body into overwork.

BRITTLE BONE DISEASE (OSTEOPOROSIS)

Brittle bone disease affects many women in the years after the menopause. Its causes are not clear, but in orthodox medicine they are seen as an interplay between inadequate calcium in the diet, too much dietary protein (which may increase excretion of calcium in the urine), and hormonal changes.

The main result is a lack of the calcium needed to maintain strong, healthy, resilient bones. After 15-20 years of poor calcium supply, the bones - especially of the lower back and hips - become weak and painful, and snap easily.

Orthodox medical studies have shown a strong correlation between this problem and an early menopause (40 years of age or before). There is also a similar link between brittle bone disease and the sudden reduction in levels of the female hormone oestrogen, after surgical removal of the ovaries. Hormone replacement therapy (see p.170) can help to avoid brittle bone disease, but it may increase the risk of other conditions. Natural therapies can avoid the need for HRT, and bring improved health.

Causes and factors

From the viewpoint of Chinese medicine, the skeleton's health and resilience relate to the body's supplies of "water energy" (see p.171). As this declines during the menopause, the bones weaken and stiffen - but only in some women. Those affected fall into two categories, as follows.

Under-used bones Any part of the body that falls into disuse eventually atrophies. Muscles which are not exercised regularly become shrunken, and flabby. Under-used bones also respond in this way to lack of use. A recent study of menopausal women in North America showed that a course of vigorous exercise, lasting one hour each day for a year, increased bone calcium level by up to one third.

A daily exercise session is therefore a simple and natural way to overcome brittle bone disease - but it must begin well before the menopause. If osteoporosis has already become a serious problem, it is advisable to consult a practitioner of natural medicine.

Decline of water energy As explained on p.171, water energy relates to the source of still, calm spiritual energy. Overwork and exhaustion deplete water energy, especially when you use willpower to drive your body too hard. The water energy can be replenished by contacting your inner source of stillness and calm.

Paradoxically, bones can be strengthened not only by vigorous exercise, but also by regular relaxation and meditation. The ideal programme is therefore one of invigorating exercise followed by relaxation and stillness.

For example, the Strong or Dynamic routine (see p.78) will help to maintain calcium levels in your bones; follow this with a relaxation or meditation session (about 20-30 minutes). If you have not exercised for some time, begin with the Weak routine and work toward the Strong routine.

Diet

- Eat fresh, high-calcium foods.
- Do not eat excessive amounts of protein, particularly animal protein, since this may encourage your body to lose calcium.

173

HYSTERECTOMY

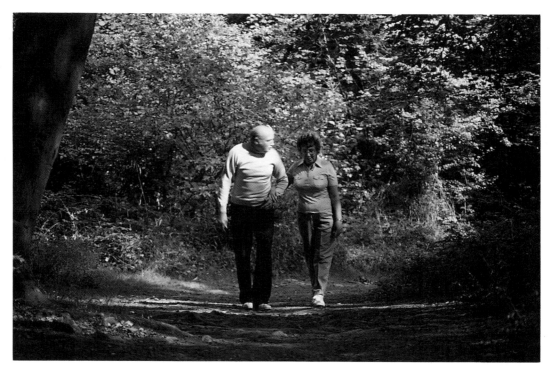

Hysterectomy is the surgical removal of the uterus (womb). Most disorders of the uterus are functional, and not a threat to life. However, conditions occasionally occur which are very serious, such as exceptionally heavy periods, fibroids, or cancer. These can develop at any time, but they are more common at and after the menopause, as energy fades from the reproductive system.

To prepare for a hysterectomy, take herbs or homeopathic remedies that direct energy to the reproductive system, such as Raspberry leaf pills (*Rubus idaeus*), for three months both before and after the operation.

Emotional reactions A hysterectomy is now such a routine, straightforward operation that many surgeons recommend it without consideration of the

Support is invaluable when an important life change takes place. A partner or friend can help to give a wider perspective.

emotions it provokes, or its later physical effects. It is quite natural to feel both fearful and angry at the thought of an important organ being removed, especially one so intimately connected with womanhood. These feelings are often countered by a strong sense of relief at the thought of curing a long-standing problem. But the fear and anger should not be ignored. Some hospitals provide a counselling service; or seek sympathetic support elsewhere, from your family physician or local adviser.

After-effects of hysterectomy A hysterectomy may bring relief from debilitating symptoms, but it rarely cures underlying

TREATMENT FOR AFTER-EFFECTS OF HYSTERECTOMY

Herbs

Note: See p.38 for doses and cautions for herbs.
● For depression, combine 2-3 herbs from this list: Echinacea (*Echinacea purpurea*), Black root (*Leptandra virginica*), Berberis (*Berberis vulgaris*), and Dandelion root (*Taraxacum officinale*).
● If the operation scar is slow to heal, or if there are internal adhesions, add St John's wort (*Hypericum perfoliatum*) and Beth root (*Trillium pendulum*) to the above prescription.

Homeopathy

Note: See p.54 for doses and cautions for homeopathic remedies.
    For depression:
● If you have mid-morning weakness and a profusion of ideas and plans - Sulphur.
● If you are emotionally volatile, with compulsive actions - Lachesis.
● If you have putrid discharges and bad breath - Kreasotum, and consult a practitioner.
● If you hold grudges and feel utter black despair - Nit. ac.
● If you experience hot flushes (hot flashes) after hysterectomy, the treatment of choice is homeopathy. Try one of the following remedies, 1 dose daily: Lachesis 12X, Aconite 6X, or Ars. alb. 30X.

imbalances. For example, if you suffer from the "hot" patterns of illness (see p.27), surgery is unlikely to change this. As periods cease, manifestations of heat - especially hot flushes (hot flashes) - may be aggravated.

Surgery may remove only the uterus, leaving the ovaries. As a result, many women experience the symptoms of a normal menstrual cycle, even though menstruation itself cannot take place. Menstruation is a time when the body clears out impurities, in preparation for new input of energy (see p.88). If the periods stop, you no longer have this outlet. Therefore, "full" patterns of illness may become more marked after the operation, since impurities that would have been discharged with the period must now be metabolized in a different way. This can make you feel very upset and emotional, even depressed. A counsellor can help you overcome these feelings and transform them into a positive attitude.

However, hysterectomy is likely to improve "weak" patterns of illness (see p.93). If periods stop, so does the loss of vital blood and body fluids.

OTHER CONDITIONS AT THE MENOPAUSE

Many changes take place at the menopause, including:
■ dry eyes and visual disturbances,
■ vaginal bleeding, dryness, irritation, or infection,
■ urinary incontinence,
■ changes in libido, and
■ joint pains.
Limited space means we cannot deal with all of them. However, they can nearly always be helped by natural and/or orthodox medicine. Consult a practitioner for further advice.

MIGRAINE

Migraine is a severe form of headache. Typically, there is a tight or boring pain, often behind the eye, and the feeling of a tight, constricting band around the head. The central feature of a migraine headache, which distinguishes it from most other types of headaches, is that it is one-sided. (In fact the term *migraine* is an abbreviation of "he*mi-cran*ial.") In severe cases there is nausea and vomiting, and visual disturbances.

Migraines affect both women and men, and they can occur at any time. But they are more common among women, and their onset is often linked to the menstrual cycle. Often the sufferer will "know" several hours in advance that a migraine headache is developing.

Internal factors

Energy factors In Chinese medicine, pain is due to obstructed energy flow. This is particularly true of migraine, which is a major symptom of energy blockage. Characteristically, migraines become

CAUTION

Several potentially serious health problems can cause migraine-like headaches. These include:
- glaucoma,
- abscess on the brain,
- inflammation of the brain (encephalitis) or its surrounding membranes (meningitis), and
- high blood pressure.

Confirm with your doctor that you are not suffering from one of these conditions, before considering treatment for migraine.

more likely when other factors slow down the normal flow of energy around the body, such as just before the period, or at a time of great stress and anxiety.

Relationship with the liver The organ most involved with free flow of energy in the body is the liver. All migraines depend to some extent on poor liver function at the vital energy level. The headache usually occurs somewhere along one of the energy channels relating to the liver, such as just behind the eye. (In Chinese medicine, the eye and liver have strong connections.) However, since migraines are generally a sign of problems at the energy level, not the physical one, orthodox medical tests of liver function are unlikely to detect anything unusual.

Someone suffering a bad migraine often feels "poisoned" because, in effect, the liver is doing a "spring-clean." The toxins which have accumulated since the last migraine are being released into the blood for processing and disposal, so that detoxification can take place. This purification also occurs around the time of the period (see p.88).

Causes in life

Diet Some migraines are due to food allergy. The "famous five" culprits are coffee, chocolate, cheese, oranges, and seafoods such as prawns and oysters. Red wine, especially the poor quality wine to which sulphur is added for preparation and storage, is another. So if you suffer from migraines, avoid these foods. Some people do not notice any link between their diet and the onset of migraines. Yet still avoid "trigger foods," since there could be long-term toxin accumulation, which may worsen the problem.

A rich diet including fried and fatty foods, and roast meats, also strains the liver. Therefore, eat a simple, easily-digested diet, and take a plate of fresh raw vegetables each day. This helps to move your energy and expel toxins.

Emotional causes On the emotional level, women are relatively stronger than men (see p.16). As a result, emotional disturbances produce reactions at the physical and vital energy levels much more quickly in women (this is one reason why migraines are more common in women). Emotions likely to trigger migraine include those which interfere with normal energy flow, for example, anger, frustration, and anxiety, when strong feelings are aroused but have no outlet.

Relationship to the menstrual cycle Some women regularly suffer migraines around the time of the period. In ortho-dox medicine, this is considered a hormonal problem; and it may be treated - often successfully - by taking female hormones, as in the contraceptive pill.

In natural medicine, migraine is not viewed as primarily a hormonal problem; more emphasis is put on life causes. The headaches may occur at any time during the cycle, but they are due to stress and accumulated toxins from the previous weeks. Nevertheless, the hormonal cycle is still involved, since it superimposes a rhythmical fluctuation on the flow of energy. Just before the period, energy flows so slowly that it can easily become obstructed (see also PMS, p.90).

Stress and lack of exercise Even with the frantic pace of modern life, some people feel that they are not doing enough. They persistently push for more. Activity is not necessarily bad, since life is short, and why not taste as many of its delights as possible? However, problems arise when this continuous effort, every day of every week, becomes a chore. Energy stagnates, and migraine is one result.

To overcome a nervous and stressful life, take regular and rhythmic exercise. Activities such as walking in the park or countryside, or easy swimming, do not push or force your energy circulation. They encourage it to flow at its own speed. Try to spend half an hour each day (more when work or family commit-ments allow) taking this kind of exercise. (Treatments are described on p.178.)

Patterns of migraine

These symptoms are common to most types of migraines:
- a tight pain on one side of your head,
- pain just behind or above one eye, and
- nausea or vomiting.

Tension pattern In this pattern, additional symptoms occur:
- the headache is accompanied by visual disturbances, flickering lights, or the world "swims" before your eyes,
- the pain is worse in bright light,
- the migraine is more likely to develop before or on the first day of your period,
- it is also triggered by tension, and
- you generally have enough energy to live your life, without undue fatigue.

Exhaustion pattern This type of migraine involves these symptoms:
- the migraine develops when you relax, such as at the weekend or on vacation,
- it is more common after your period,
- you have a pale face, and
- you often feel worn down and tired.

TREATMENT FOR MIGRAINE

Herbs

Note: See p.38 for doses and cautions for herbs.
- Feverfew (*Chrysanthemum parthenium*), available in various forms, is helpful for many patterns of migraine.

For tension pattern:
- Take the relaxants Valerian (*Valeriana officinalis*), Motherwort (*Leonurus cardiaca*), and Feverfew (*Chrysanthemum parthenium*) together, for up to three months.
- Use Mugwort (*Artemisia vulgaris*), Wormwood (*Artemisia absinthum*), Tansy (*Artemisia tanacetum*), or Angelica (*Angelica arcangelica*), as a replacement for Feverfew.

For exhaustion pattern:
- Take herbs for at least 3 months as an adjunct to strengthening energy. Select Gentian (*Gentiana lutea*), Berberis (*Berberis vulgaris*), Black cohosh (*Cimicifuga racemosa*), and Water lily (*Nymphaea alba*), combined with Feverfew. Gentian and Berberis are tonics, Black cohosh aids the female hormones, and Water lily cools the uterus.

Homeopathy

Note: See p.54 for doses and cautions for homeopathic remedies. Take the remedy at 6X potency 3 times daily, or more infrequently at higher potencies (see p.56). Some remedies may provoke a migraine at first, but do not be discouraged. Otherwise, take them as soon as the pain starts.

For tension pattern:
- If you are restless, and angry much of the time, the pain pulsates, and one cheek is hot - Chamomilla.
- If you are easily excited or frightened, the pain comes from the nape of your neck, and you have thick nasal mucus - Gelsemium.
- If you are very tense and cannot sleep - Coffea.
- If you feel emotionally drained, you cannot bear tobacco smoke, and the pain is like a nail being driven into your skull - Ignatia.

For exhaustion pattern:
- If you have difficulty showing your emotions, and the bursting headache arrives with your period - Sepia.
- If you are thin and pale, with an intense disposition, and long-lasting headaches - Silica.
- If you are emotional and tearful, and have headaches after study - Pulsatilla.

Exercises

Note: See p.70 for details of exercise routines. Start exercises gently; if you are too vigorous, this could provoke migraine.
- All twist-type exercises are beneficial. They include Lizard, Temple guardian, Wall twist, and Mermaid.
- Film director, in any chair with arms. Sit with your left leg crossed over your right. Hold the chair's left arm with both hands. Exhaling, pull yourself around, looking over your left shoulder; hold for 30 seconds. Exhale and face the front. Cross your legs the other way and repeat in the opposite direction.

Neck exercises are important for migraine. As well as Neck roll (see p.81), practise these:
- Bend your neck slowly forward, chin toward your breastbone. Then bend your neck slowly back as far as you can, with jaws loose. Bend forward again, then back again but with closed jaws. Repeat 10 times.
- Bend your neck and try to touch your ear to each shoulder. Repeat 10 times.
- Keeping your gaze level, rotate your head to the left and right, as far as you can. Repeat 10 times.

Naturopathy

- Evening primrose oil and vitamin B complex supplements may bring relief from migraine.

CYSTITIS

Cystitis is inflammation of the bladder, usually caused by infecting bacteria. It is characterized by dull aching or soreness in the bladder region, a pressing sensation in the lower abdomen, an almost uncontrollable urge to urinate, and then burning or scalding sensations upon passing urine.

This physically awkward and socially embarrassing condition is also potentially dangerous. There is a risk of the infection spreading up the urinary tract to the kidneys, causing the more serious disease of nephritis. For this reason, cystitis may well be treated with broad-spectrum antibiotics. Recurrent attacks should be investigated by a physician.

Causes

The most common sources of infection are from your own anal region, from swimming places with bacteria in the water, and through sexual intercourse, either when bacteria that are harmless to one person are transmitted to the partner, or through physical bruising of the urethral area.

You can considerably reduce the risk of infection by developing the habit of promptly visiting the lavatory and urinating immediately after swimming or sexual intercourse. This flushes any hostile bacteria from the urethra. Also, pay scrupulous attention to hygiene.

DANGER SIGNS

Bleeding from the urethra may signify a more serious problem, such as an ulcer, polyps, or cancer. Seek urgent help from your physician.

Composition of the urine The bacteria involved in cystitis are often very common ones. In these cases, the composition of the urine causes the problem. Urine should normally be completely sterile, and bacteria should not be able to multiply in it. If your urine composition alters, however, the bacteria can thrive and cause inflammation.

In natural medicine, the liver rather than the kidney is the main organ controlling urine composition. The liver breaks down toxins that accumulate in your body. The kidneys filter the waste products, but these will be very concentrated if the liver is not working well, and any bacteria can therefore thrive on the excretions. This leads to the acid urine pattern of cystitis.

Energy flow A healthy body has the ability to fight off infection, but this needs energy. So if an infection takes hold, this means your normal flow of energy has been disrupted. This can happen if you hold on when your bladder is full, or wear underclothing that is too tight, preventing normal circulation of energy, or have very frequent sexual intercourse, or sit still for too long without physical exercise. Deficiency of energy stems from causes in everyday life (see p.25).

Patterns of cystitis

In the acute pattern, symptoms are pronounced and clear, but short-lived. In the weak or chronic pattern, symptoms come and go over a longer period and may be punctuated by acute attacks.

Symptoms of the acute pattern are:
■ soreness in bladder,
■ you have a great desire to urinate, but pass only a few drops,

TREATMENT FOR CYSTITIS

• Drink lots of water, which helps to dilute the acids in the urine.
• Take 1 level teaspoonful of bicarbonate of soda, to neutralize acids in the urine.
• Eat as much parsley as you can.
• Avoid red meat, spices, and alcohol.

Herbs

Note: See p.38 for doses and cautions for herbs.
    For all patterns:
• Buchu (*Barosma betulina*), Cleavers (*Galium aparine*), and Horsetails (*Equisetum arvensis*). Take one-quarter of a 5mls teaspoon of tincture of each herb, sipped in warm water, every 2-4 hours.
• If there is bleeding, add Tormentil (*Potentilla tormentilla*) or Shepherd's purse (*Capsella bursa-pastoris*).

• Other herbs that cool the urinary passage are Plantain (*Plantago lanceolata*) and Marshmallow (*Althea officinalis*), best taken as a syrup or tea made from fresh or dried herb.
• For the acid urine pattern, add Valerian (*Valeriana officinalis*) and Fringe tree (*Chionanthus virginica*).
    For the weak pattern:
• Sweet sumach (*Rhus aromatica*), Beth root (*Trillium pendulum*), Horsetails (*Equisetum arvensis*), and Hydrangea (*Hydrangea aborescens*), 20 drops of tincture of each herb in water, 3 times daily.

Homeopathy

Note: See p.54 for doses and cautions for homeopathic remedies.
    For all patterns:
• If you have strong burning pains, great thirst, and a strong sex drive - Cantharis.

• If you also have digestive disturbances - Berberis.
• If the pain is more pricking, and you have fluid retention but no great thirst - Apis mel.
• If the pain burns, but you feel otherwise chilly - Capsicum.
    For the weak pattern:
• If you have an ache in the kidneys and a stronger ache in the bladder - Equisetum.
• If the pain in the bladder and urethra becomes worse after exposure to cold - Dulcamara.
• If you have to wait while the urine starts, and it flows slowly - Hepar sulph.
• If you also have stress incontinence - Causticum.

Exercises

Note: See p.70 for details of exercise routines.
• Pelvic energizer (see p.104).
• The Great pull (see p.111).

■ pain on urinating, and
■ a temporary improvement afterward.
    Symptoms of the acid urine pattern are:
■ the urine feels scalding, and seems to burn the skin wherever it remains,
■ your tongue has a yellow coat,
■ you feel irritable and impatient,
■ you have indigestion, but feel better after vigorous exercise, and
■ spicy foods, red meat, or alcohol make the problem worse.

    Symptoms of the weak pattern include the following:
■ an ache in the bladder, which tends to come and go,
■ the ache is worse after urinating, and
■ you feel generally exhausted.

Parsley is a time-honoured remedy for cystitis. Eat it preferably as a fresh garnish, chopped or grated, or as a culinary flavouring. Dried parsley is less effective.

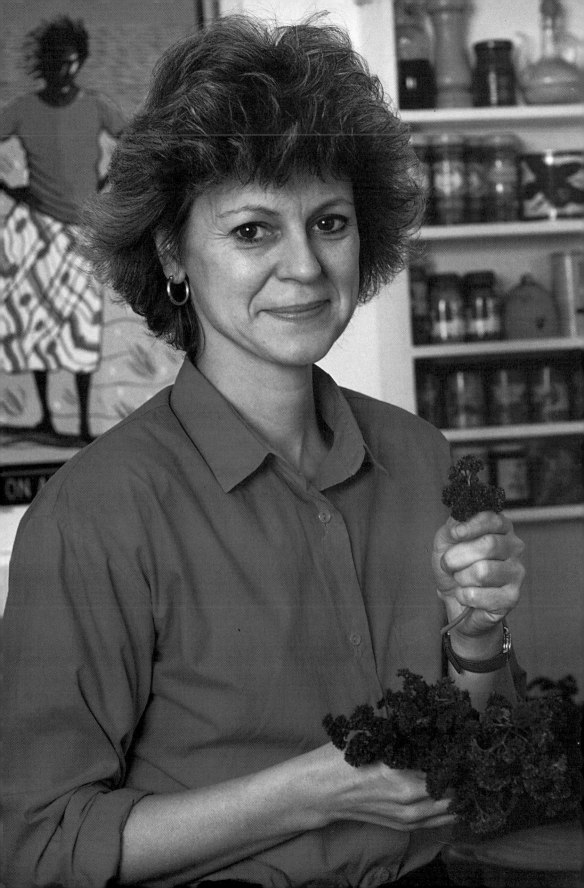

CONTRACEPTION

Enjoying lovemaking, without the worry of bringing a new life into the world, is an age-old problem. Conception is a natural outcome of making love, and any attempt to thwart nature is bound to bring problems.

Physical methods The most straightforward method of contraception is to place a physical barrier in the path of the sperm. Today, we can choose from various methods such as condoms or caps which have few, if any, side-effects on health. However, many couples dislike using them. Such methods can interfere with the natural rhythm of lovemaking, making it seem premeditated and calculated, and disturbing the spontaneous expression of tenderness and passion.

Contraceptive pill For a new life to begin, a ripe egg, or ovum, is necessary. The contraceptive pill changes the natural hormonal cycle to prevent ripening and release (ovulation) of an egg. But the various types of pill have side-effects, which can be understood by taking a closer look at what they do in the body.

Female hormones are not merely chemical regulators. They are intimately related to mood and feelings. Anything that interferes with hormones also disturbs moods and emotions. This is particularly true of the contraceptive pill, when the effect of artificially regulating the cycle can be to deaden emotional response. The effect is more pronounced in some women - they become less responsive, and possibly even seriously depressed.

Hormonal suppression has its counterpart on the energy level. Energy circulation slows down, which can lead to an accumulation of toxins. In general, older women are affected more. The level of emotional energy diminishes with age, so that the deadening effect of oral contraception is greater at 40 years of age, for example, than at 20.

What are the pill's long-term effects? There are medical risks such as raised blood pressure, thrombosis (blood clots), problems in re-establishing a regular cycle, subsequent low fertility, and even certain growths and cancers. These risks are minimized when your doctor or family planning counsellor advises the right type of pill for your own situation.

Deadened emotional responses can suppress your spirit, and cause accumulation of toxins on the physical level. Your true individuality and personality have difficulty in finding full expression, and increased toxins may make the physical body more prone to ailments.

Intra-uterine contraceptive device The IUCD (IUD or "coil") is a shaped solid object, usually with traces of copper, which is inserted into the uterus to prevent pregnancy. The exact mechanism is still not understood. But it is said that in natural medicine, inserting a foreign body into the uterus causes local stagnation of energy. When the energy cannot circulate normally, there is never enough available for a foetus to develop. The side-effects of the IUCD are also readily explained by stagnation of energy in the womb area (see opposite).

Rhythm methods The normal cycle allows only a few days of fertility, around the time that the egg is released - normally about 14 days after the period starts. For most of the remainder of the cycle, the cervix, or neck of the uterus, is effectively closed by a plug of viscous mucus.

The fibres of the mucus align transversely across the cervical canal, to form a barrier. As ovulation approaches, the mucus becomes thinner and less viscous, and the fibres align lengthwise along the canal, allowing sperm to pass.

The principle of the rhythm method is to make love only during infertile times. However, this has three main drawbacks.

First, the egg can be fertilized for two or three days after its release. No intercourse must take place until these days have elapsed, which may be awkward.

Second, sperm can live for up to four days, so no intercourse must take place for four days before ovulation, either. If you have irregular periods, ovulation can be hard to predict.

Third, there may be another fertile time, which is not generally recognized. This is when the moon is in the same position in the sky as it was when the woman was born. If you are sceptical of astrology, such an idea seems preposterous. However, recent research is revealing how the moon influences the bodily cycles of both women and men. It seems that, although a woman normally produces only one egg per cycle, if she has intercourse at this very sensitive time, this can stimulate one ovary to release another egg. This ability to release an egg "on demand" is well known among animals.

Guidelines for making a choice

Each method of contraception has its advantages and disadvantages. Mechanical techniques tend to interrupt the normal flow of lovemaking; chemical methods interfere with the emotions and block creative energy, thereby opening the way for other problems; the rhythm

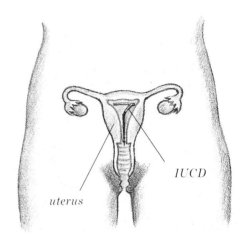

The IUCD may have several side-effects, such as menstrual cramps, endometriosis, ectopic pregnancies, risk of infection, and subsequent low fertility - explained by energy stagnation.

method requires good organization and practical application. So which method should you use?

The first part of the answer is to consult with your partner, orthodox physician, and practitioner of natural medicine, to discuss the pros and cons as they relate to your own health and attitudes. You should then be able to decide on the second part of the answer.

The pill is the most effective method, and extremely widely used, but it works against natural body physiology by suppressing the normal cycle. During later years, when emotional energy wanes, the liver is less able to metabolize impurities in the system, and the risks of contraceptive pills therefore become greater.

If you have a stable relationship, investigate the retention of semen method. This is difficult to master, but it can bring lasting contentment (see Resources, p.186).

THE HOME NATURAL MEDICINE CHEST

Most households have a cupboard some-where for pills, ointments, sticking plasters, and similar items. As you become interested in natural medicines, it is worthwhile building up a basic stock of commonly-used remedies.

As explained on p.10, most people find that they are instinctively drawn to one type of natural therapy, such as herbs, or homeopathy. (Other types of natural therapies include tissue salts, Bach flower remedies, and naturopathic remedies, see p.186.) The basic medicine chest provides a good starting point from which you can explore your use of natural remedies, and the ways they affect you. Then, as you progress, you can stock more of the types of remedies with which you feel comfortable. Remember that the therapeutic exercises and massages may also be used in combination with either natural remedies or orthodox medicines.

The medicine chest should be in a convenient place and readily accessible, even in the middle of the night, but it should be inaccessible to children.

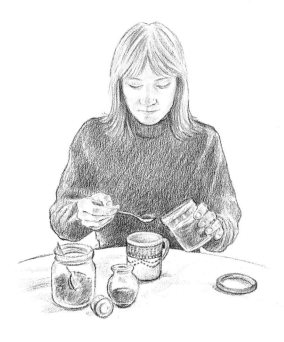

Most herbal teas are made by infusing the fresh herb in boiling water. However, some herbs have very volatile ingredients, so use hot water. Refer to the Materia Medica, pp.42-53, for details. Different herbs may be combined for cumulative effects.

HOMEOPATHIC REMEDIES

Note: See p.54 for doses and cautions for homeopathic remedies. Stock 6X potencies at first.

The following remedies are particularly wide-acting, and they are useful to keep on hand for all manner of problems:
- Aconite.
- Arnica
- Ars. alb.
- Belladonna

- Carbo veg.
- Gelsemium.
- Lycopodium.
- Mag. phos.
- Merc. sol.
- Nat. mur.
- Nux vom.
- Phosphorus.
- Pulsatilla.
- Silica.
- Sulphur.

These further remedies are generally specific for

women's problems, although some have more wide-ranging therapeutic uses:
- Actea racemosa.
- Apis
- Borax.
- Calc. carb.
- Cantharis.
- Caulophyllum.
- Chamomilla.
- Ignatia.
- Lachesis.
- Sepia.

HERBAL REMEDIES

Note: See page 38 for doses and cautions for herbs.

If you obtain all the herbs mentioned in this book, you may find that you never use some of them. This selection provides a few key indications, to guide you in your choice.

Herbs for general use

- Yarrow (*Achillea mille-folium*) is a tonic that regulates periods and helps influenza.
- Fringe tree (*Chionanthus virginica*) aids liver problems.
- Echinacea (*Echinacea purpurea*) soothes spots, boils, and rashes.
- Gentian (*Gentiana lutea*) is a stomach tonic.
- Licorice (*Glycyrrhiza glabra*) acts as a general tonic and "pick-me-up."
- Golden seal (*Hydrastis canadensis*) is a digestive tonic that clears chronic mucus (phlegm or catarrh).
- Butternut *(Juglans cinerea)* is a laxative.
- Hops (*Humulus lupulus*) soothes and relaxes muscles and nerves.
- St John's wort (*Hypericum perfoliatum*) relaxes, and heals wounds.
- Black root (*Leptandra virginica*) tonifies the liver.
- Lobelia (*Lobelia inflata*) soothes cramps and coughs.
- Chamomile (*Matricaria chamomilla*) is a relaxant, especially for insomnia.
- Catmint (*Nepeta cataria*) brings down fevers.
- White poplar (*Populus tremuloides*) is a tonic, especially for lower body.
- Cascara (*Rhamnus purshiana*) is a laxative.
- Sage (*Salvia officinalis*) is a useful all-round herb.
- Lime (*Tilia europea*), commonly available as tea bags, makes a relaxing drink that soothes fevers.
- Valerian (*Valeriana officinalis*) is a general relaxant and encourages sleep.

Herbs for women's problems

- Mugwort (*Artemisia vulgaris*) regulates periods.
- Marigold petals (*Calendula officinalis*) stop bleeding in "hot" pattern ailments (see p.27).
- Blue cohosh (*Caulophyllum thalactroides*) relieves tension and menstrual cramps.
- False unicorn root (*Chamaelirium luteum*) helps pelvic weakness and uterine prolapse.
- Feverfew (*Chrysanthemum parthenium*) treats migraine .
- Black cohosh (*Cimicifuga racemosa*) aids pelvic weakness and cramps.
- Lady's slipper (*Cypripedium pubescens*) is a strong relaxant.
- Wild yam (*Dioscorea villosa*) regulates periods.
- Motherwort (*Leonurus cardiaca*) regulates periods and heart palpitations.
- Squaw vine (*Mitchella repens*) and Beth root (*Trillium pendulum*) are useful for pelvic weakness and prolapse.
- Nettles (*Urtica dioica*) fortify against anaemia.
- Cramp bark (*Viburnum opulus*) soothes menstrual cramps.
- Chaste tree (*Vitex agnus castus*) regulates the female hormones.

Culinary herbs

- Dill seeds (*Anethum graveolens*) and Fennel seeds (*Foeniculum vulgare*) are stomach tonics.

Cystitis

- Keep the following herbs - Buchu (*Barosma betulina*), Horsetails (*Equisetum arvensis*), Cleavers (*Galium aparine*), Cranesbill (*Geranium maculatum*), and Corn silk (*Zea mays*).

Heavy periods

- Keep the following remedies - Shepherd's purse (*Capsella bursa pastoris*), Cranesbill (*Geranium maculatum*), and Tormentil (*Potentilla tormentilla*).

RESOURCES

Further reading

There are many excellent books on specific aspects of women's health problems. Some titles are regularly updated, so try to obtain the most recent edition.

Herbs

● *The Illustrated Herbal Handbook*, Juliette de Baracli Levy, Faber & Faber
● *Culpeper's Complete Herbal*, Nicholas Culpeper (various publishers)
● *A Modern Herbal*, Mrs Grieve, Penguin
● *The Herb Book*, John Lust, Bantam
● *The Complete New Herbal*, ed Richard Mabey, Penguin (UK), and as *The New Age Herbalist,* Collier Books (US)
● *Natural Healing in Gynaecology*, Rina Nissim, Pandora
● *Wise Woman Childbearing Year*, Susun Weed, Ashtree New York

Homeopathy

● *Pocket Manual of Materia Medica with Repertory*, Boericke (various publishers)
● *Everybody's Guide to Homeopathic Medicines*, Dr M Panos & J Heimlich
● *Homeopathic Medicine: A Doctor's Guide*, Dr Trevor Smith
● *Homeopathic Remedies for Women's Ailments*, Phyllis Speight, Health Science Press (CW Daniel)
● *The Natural Family Doctor,* ed Dr Andrew Stanway, Century Hutchinson (UK), Simon and Schuster (US)

Alexander technique

● *The Alexander Technique*, Liz Hodgkinson, Piatkus Press

Bach remedies

● *The 12 Healers*, Dr E Bach, CW Daniel
● *Bach Flower Therapy: Theory and Practice*, M Scheffer, Thorsons

Diet and ailments

● *Clear Body, Clear Mind,* Leon Chaitow, Unwin Hyman (UK), and as *The Body/Mind Purification Program,* Simon and Schuster (US)
● *Eating and Allergy*, Robert Eagle, Thorsons
● *Food Combining for Health*, Doris Grant and Jean Joice, Thorsons
● *Good Food Gluten Free*, Hilda Cherry Hills, Roberts Publications, London
● *The Food Combining Cookbook*, Edwina Lidolt, Thorsons
● *Diet for Common Ailments,* Penny Stanway, Sidgwick and Jackson (UK & Australia), and as *Foods for Common Ailments,* Simon and Schuster (US)
● *Beat PMT Through Diet*, M Stewart, Ebury Park Books

Women's books

● *Natural Pregnancy*, Janet Balaskas, Sidgwick and Jackson (UK), Interlink (US), Simon and Schuster (Australia)
● *Billings Method of Family Planning*, Dr E Billings, Thorsons
● *The New Our Bodies Ourselves*, The Boston Women's Health Book Collective, Penguin Books
● *Ourselves, Growing Older*, The Boston Women's Health Book Collective, Fontana/Collins
● *The Natural Birth Control Book*, Art Rosenblum, Aquarian Research Foundation, Philadelphia
● *Alternative Maternity*, Nicky Wesson, Optima

Exercise

● *The Way of Energy,* Master Lam Kam Chuen, Gaia Books (UK), Simon and Schuster (US, Australia)
● *Yoga for Common Ailments,* R Nagarathna, H Nagendra, R Monro, Gaia Books (UK), Simon and Schuster (US), Angus and Robertson (Australia)
● *The Book of Yoga*, Siva-nanda Yoga Centre, Ebury Press (UK) and *The Siva-nanda Companion to Yoga,* Simon and Schuster (US)

Suppliers

- Susun Weed Avena Botanicals, POB 365 Rockport, ME 04856
- Equinox Botanicals Rt 1, Box 71 Rutland, OH 45775 Frontier Cooperative Herbs Rt 1, Box 31 Norway, Iowa 52318
- Herb Pharm, Box 116 Williams, OR 97544
- Iris Herbal Products, 940 Austin Ave NE, Atlanta, GA 30307
- Meadowbrook Herbs, Whispering Pines Road, Wyoming, RI 02898
- Pan's Forest Herb Co, 411 Raven's Road, Port Townsend, WA 98368
- Ryan Drum, Waldron Island, WA 98297
- Willow Rain Herb Farm, POB 15 Grubville, MO 63041
- Wish Garden Herbs, PO Box 1304, Boulder, CO 80306

Organizations and societies

- American Association of Naturopathic Physicians, Post Office Box 20386, Seattle, Washington 98102. Phone 206-323-7601
- American Holistic Medical Association and Foundation, 2002 Eastlake Avenue East, Seattle, Washington 98102. Phone 206-322-6842. (Write for details of their regular magazine)
- International Foundation for Homeopathy, 2366 Eastlake Avenue East, Suite 301, Seattle, Washington 98102. Phone 206-324-8230
- Ellon (Bach USA) Inc., PO Box 320, Woodmere, NY 11598

The following publish or review books on natural and holistic therapies:

- Eastland Press, 611 Post Avenue, Suite 3, Seattle, Washington 98104. Phone 206-587 6013
- Redwing Reviews, Redwing Book Co, 44 Linden Street, Brookline, Ma 02146. Phone 617-738-4664

INDEX

The main page reference for each major entry is printed in **bold** type. Page references to illustrations are in *italics*.

Acknowledgements

The author would like to thank: the doctors at the Nanjing College of Traditional Chinese Medicine, who were his teachers, and all of the consultants who helped so much in the production of this book.

Gaia Books would like to thank: Oriana Battistella, Anne Beach, and Claudia Cran for modelling for the illustrations; Libby Hoseason for editorial management; Sara Mathews for design and production coordination; Susan Walby and Alison Jones for production; Chris Nall for delivery services; Jane Parker for word processing and preparing the Index; Susan Berry, Richard Dawes and Philippa Underwood for editorial assistance; David Whelan for technical guidance; Doug Whitworth and Phil Gamble for printing services; Shona Wood for picture research; and Samantha Nunn.

Photographic credits

Title page Steve Janson/Life File; pages 9, 87, 95, 110 (Melrose Films), 123 Shona Wood; pages 13, 174 Mick Rock/Cephas Picture Library; pages 17, 149 Anthea Sieveking/Collections; page 19 Clive Barda; page 20 John Lambie/Ace; pages 24, 82, 181 Sandra Buchanan; page 29 Janina Struk/Format; page 35 David Johnson; page 37 Neal Street Remedies; page 129 Nancy Durrell McKenna/ Hutchison; page 135 Robert Francis / Hutchison; page 138 Gabe Palmer/Ace; page 146 Zefa; page 160 Geoff Du Feu/Ace; page 169 Chris Barry/Action Plus.

Approximate equivalents

One drop = 0.04 mls
One teacup = 8fl ozs = 250mls
One tablespoon = 15mls
One teaspoon = 5mls
One wineglass = 2fl ozs = 100mls